UPDATES IN EMERGENCY MEDICINE

UPDATES IN EMERGENCY MEDICINE

Edited by

John D. Cahill

Rhode Island Hospital
Providence, Rhode Island

Kluwer Academic / Plenum Publishers
New York, Boston, Dordrecht, London, Moscow

ISBN 0-306-47470-0

©2003 Kluwer Academic / Plenum Publishers, New York
233 Spring Street, New York, New York 10013

http://www.wkap.nl/

10 9 8 7 6 5 4 3 2 1

A C.I.P. record for this book is available from the Library of Congress

To Elizabeth Anne Stock Cahill,
who had faith that education could make a better world.

CONTRIBUTORS

David Brodkin • University of Massachusetts School of Medicine, Worcester, Massachusetts

John D. Cahill, M.D. • Assistant Professor of Community Health, Brown Medical School; Department of Emergency Medicine, Rhode Island Hospital; and Department of Infectious Diseases, The Miriam Hospital, Providence, Rhode Island

Scott J. Cohen, M.D. • Director, Global Pediatric Alliance, Oakland, California

Scott Durgin, M.D. • Department of Emergency Medicine, Rhode Island Hospital, Providence, Rhode Island

Deirdre M. Fearon, Ed.M., M.D. • Department of Pediatrics and Section of Emergency Medicine, Brown Medical School; and Pediatric Emergency Medicine, Hasbro Children's Hospital, Providence, Rhode Island

Daren Girard, M.D. • Assistant Professor of Medicine, Brown University; and Department of Emergency Medicine, The Miriam Hospital, Providence, Rhode Island

Robert Partridge, M.D., M.P.H. • Assistant Professor of Medicine, Brown Medical School; and Department of Emergency Medicine, Rhode Island Hospital, Providence, Rhode Island

Lawrence Proano, M.D. • Associate Professor, Brown University/Rhode Island Hospital, Department of Emergency Medicine, Providence, Rhode Island

James Pyskaty, M.D. • Assistant Director, Global Pediatric Alliance, Oakland, California

Walter N. Simmons, M.D., M.P.H. • Fellow in Emergency Medicine, Brown University, Providence, Rhode Island

Robert H. Woolard, M.D. • Associate Professor of Medicine, Chief of Section of Emergency Medicine, Brown Medical School, Providence, Rhode Island

PREFACE

Since the beginning of mankind, medical emergencies have existed. However, only in the last several decades has the specialty of emergency medicine developed. The United States and the United Kingdom were probably the first to recognize the need for a physician to be properly trained in this discipline. It quickly became evident that many lives could be saved by physicians trained in this art. Now is an exciting time for the field, as more and more countries have recognized this and are developing training programs in emergency medicine.

This book is based upon a course in emergency medicine that was held in Ireland in the fall of 2001 and on several other lectures given that year. The course was held at the Royal College of Surgeons in Ireland and was a joint effort of faculty comprised from the Brown University program in Emergency Medicine, Providence, Rhode Island and Beaumont Hospital, Dublin, Ireland. The goals of the course were to introduce the basic principles and practice of emergency medicine, to present some cutting edge topics, and to help encourage an interest in developing an academic training program in emergency medicine in Ireland.

I hope that this collection of papers will be enjoyed by: medical students, residents, attending physicians, and by all who pursue an interest in emergency medicine. It is not intended to be a comprehensive text on emergency medicine. The purpose is to present some pertinent topics and observations from experienced physicians in a scientific and evidence-based fashion.

A special thanks to the Ireland Funds who generously provided a grant to make this all possible, to all my colleagues who generously donated their time to lecture, and to Mr. Shelby Coffey III and Dr. Mary Lee Coffey.

John D. Cahill MD

ACKNOWLEDGMENTS

The course on Updates in Emergency Medicine from which this book is based, would not have been possible without the efforts of the following individuals: Dr. John D. Cahill II, Mr. Shelby Coffey III, Dr. Mary Lee Coffey, Mr. Ben Bradlee, Senator Maurice Hayes & the Ireland Funds, Professor Kevin O'Malley & the Royal College of Surgeons in Ireland, Dr. Kevin M Cahill, and Mr. Aidan Gleeson. This book would not have been possible without the help of Mr. Aaron Johnson at Kluwer Academic/Plenum Publishers, Ms. Laurie Bjornson, and all the authors who kindly contributed their time and efforts.

CONTENTS

THE EVALUATION OF CARDIAC CHEST PAIN AND EQUIVALENT SYNDROMES IN THE EMERGENCY DEPARTMENT

Robert H. Woolard, M.D. [*]

Therapeutic and diagnostic advances have continued to reduce mortality and morbidity from acute coronary syndrome. Thrombolytic therapy and numerous other medical and invasive options are now widely available for treatment of acute myocardial infarction (MI). Bedside enzymatic assays and cardiac imaging modalities are more available for rapid diagnosis.

Education campaigns concerning the benefits of early intervention in MI have been launched with the hope of influencing the public and medical communities. Chest Pain centers have been opened and the public, legal and medical expectation for immediate therapy has now become routine. The emergency physician is more able than ever to meet this expectation for immediate treatment. Unfortunately, patient delay, EMS (Emergency Medical Services) delay, ED delay and systems factors may limit delivery.

Public education campaigns have focused on patient delay prior to 911 calls. On average, patients wait more than 2 hours from onset of symptoms before placing a call for help. In spite of numerous public education campaigns, patients are just becoming aware of the benefits of early intervention. Transport time of the EMS is estimated to average from 7 to 22 minutes. A large proportion of prehospital delay must be attributed to patient recognition and action. Because some individuals wait many hours to days before seeking medical care for symptoms, mean delay times are significantly longer than median delay times in all reported studies. A variety of factors have been associated with delay times. These findings have often been inconsistent across studies, perhaps due to different study populations, methods of data collection, or definitions. The literature suggests that sudden onset pain is associated with shorter delay times, and older age, female gender, and African-American race are associated with longer delay times. History of prior MI does not decrease delay times. The presence of angina either has no effect or is associated with longer delay time. Both chronic stable angina and angina

---

[*] Robert Woolard M.D., Associate Professor of Medicine, Chief of Section of Emergency Medicine at Brown Medical School, Providence, Rhode Island

increasing in severity are associated with longer delay times. Education level has not been associated with delay time. Consulting with a spouse or unrelated individuals is associated with significant higher delay times, as is consulting with a physician. Finally, self-treatment for symptoms results in a significant delay. Patients with known coronary disease are less likely to seek evaluation early, even when they experience new and different symptoms.

EMS delays might be overcome by thrombolytic therapy in the field. The MITI (Myocardial Infarction Triage and Intervention) trial showed that prehospital thrombolytic therapy given by paramedics did not offer any measurable advantage over the improved ED efficiency realized during the study. Thrombolytic therapy was accomplished within 20 minutes of patient arrival at the ED. The current national guidelines promote a 30 minute "door to drug" and 60 minute "door to cath lab" time through the ED. There is growing enthusiasm for primary angioplasty in the USA. Throughout the TIMI (Thrombolysis in Myocardial Infarction) trials, US researchers lamented the low numbers of patients treated within the first hour of their symptoms. In a report of the prehospital study group, 8 prominent hospitals spread over the US revealed that the average time from 911 call to ED arrival was 46 minutes and the time from ED arrival to thrombolytic therapy was 84 minutes. Over the next few years, more patients may begin to seek attention early in the course of their initial episodes of symptomatic coronary artery disease (CAD), prehospital ECG and other efforts to improve efficiency may reduce delays.

The emergency physician is challenged to make the diagnosis of MI quickly and accurately. In the US, missed myocardial infarction (MI) represents the greatest source of malpractice loss in emergency medicine. Largely for this reason, the first clinical care guideline developed by ACEP (American College of emergency Physicians) concerned the management of CP. The public, legal, and even the cardiologist's expectation seems to be that an emergency evaluation of CP will have 100% sensitivity for Acute Coronary Syndrome (ACS). Throughout the US the threshold for admission/evaluation of CP is low. About 50% of those admitted do not have ACS.

Payers for health care may have an entirely different expectation of the evaluation. Payers want to minimize the cost of the evaluation. A much more efficient and less costly process has driven in part the development of CP centers in the US. The emergency physician's initial concern when evaluating a patient with CP is to make a diagnosis of ST segment elevation MI requiring aggressive treatment. The electrocardiogram (ECG) plays the important role as the initial test. The ECG should be obtained and interpreted promptly, within 5–10 minutes of patient arrival. The majority of patients with CP will not have diagnostic ECGs. No single diagnostic test or combination of tests has been able to achieve either 100% sensitivity or specificity. Similarly no single clinical variable can be used to exclude MI.

There are several new diagnostic avenues available to the emergency physician. Following these avenues in the evaluation of patients presenting to the ED with CP and equivalent syndromes is an area of active ongoing investigation. These avenues may make possible the more accurate detection of non ST-segment elevation MI (NSTE MI), unstable angina, and CAD earlier in the ED. To understand the strengths and limitations of present and future diagnostic tests, it is necessary to outline the basic pathophysiology. The acute ACS includes unstable angina, NSTE MI, and ST-segment elevation MI. Our current understanding is that these syndromes occur after an acute decrease in coronary blood flow. This diminution in blood flow is usually secondary to thrombosis at the site of a fissured atherosclerotic plaque. The degree of thrombosis and the severity of the acute symptoms can be modified by the many factors.

ATHEROSCLEROTIC PLAQUE

Atherosclerotic plaques are the result of chronic damage to arterial endothelial cells at discrete places in the coronary arteries. This damage leads to accumulations of lipids within the endothelial cell and monocytes in the neighboring vascular wall. This process is potentiated by vasoactive amines, high cholesterol and smoking. Once initiated, a plaque becomes self-sustaining through the release of inflammatory mediators and the proliferation of smooth muscle cells in the media of the artery. Plaques continue to grow by their interaction with the platelets and the intrinsic coagulation system through repeated cycles of fissuring and thrombosis. Plaques incorporate variable proportions of lipid, fibrin, proteinaceous material and cellular elements as they form. Hence plaques vary in growth rates and stability. In certain cases, larger plaques grow to impede blood flow to a critical level. This process is gradual resulting in infarcts that will be smaller (or even silent), since collateral circulation is developed. In other cases the rupture of a small, hemodynamically insignificant plaque leads to an acute, thrombotic occlusion of blood flow (angina and MI). The role of inflammation at the onset of plaque rupture and thrombosis is under active investigation. It is estimated that 85% of the infarct related atherosclerotic lesions are less than 75% occlusive. The current view is that small lipid rich plaques can be very unstable, whereas larger, more stenotic plaques are usually stable.

Clot formation depends on the degree of plaque disruption, the degree of stenosis, and risk factors. The thrombogenic risk varies by day of the year and hour of the day, to hour. Clot formation is influenced by circulating levels of catecholamine, cholesterol, lipoprotein A (a competitive inhibitor of fibrinolysis), factor VII and fibrinogen. To treat MI, clots can be lysed and platelet aggregation can be blocked. Vasoconstriction in response to thrombosis can be a key element in the final outcome of a clotted coronary. Factors which promote vasodilation will lessen the ensuing ischemia or infarct. The presence of intact endothelium within the coronary tree promotes vasodilation. Platelets release mediators such as serotonin and ADP which cause vasodilation in all arterial areas covered by intact endothelium. In addition, normal endothelium will release prostacyclin and factors which cause smooth muscle relaxation and inhibit platelet aggregation. Once a plaque fissures, the result will depend on a complex interaction of factors which depend on a person's genetic makeup, recent environmental circumstances, and the degree of chronic vascular disease.

PATIENT PRESENTATIONS

Most patients who have already sustained a transmural MI upon ED presentation will be properly identified by the emergency physician after taking a history and interpreting a standard 12 lead ECG. It is incumbent upon emergency physicians to be expert in the interpretation of the ECG. Data from the Framingham study suggests that as many as 25% of MIs are not recognized by the patient. Some patients do not seek medical attention for their ACS. Several large studies of CP patients have characterized their symptoms in the ED. Lee developed the following table from his large series of ED patients complaining of CP. Table one shows the proportions of patients with symptoms or signs usually considered atypical for CAD who were noted after completion of evaluation to have either MI or angina.

Table 1: Atypical signs & symptoms and correlated diagnosis

Symptoms	MI	Angina
Sharp/stabbing pain	5%	17%
Pain partially varies with respiration	6%	7%
Pain fully reproduced on palpation	5%	2%
Pain partially reproduced on palpation	6%	18%

Diaphoresis occurs in as many as half of patients with acute infarction and is a particularly useful sign when present. Dyspnea is present in about a third of all patients with acute infarction and is more common as a presenting symptom of MI in the elderly than CP. Atypical presentations such as syncope or indigestion are more common in the elderly. It is generally agreed that in the absence of signs of congestive heart failure or circulatory failure, that the physical exam adds little to the difficult diagnostic evaluations of subtle cases of acute MI.

In one of the most comprehensive studies of ED CP patients, Lee looked at 3,077 patients evaluated in the ED for CP. 1794 were admitted and 1283 discharged. 26% of patients admitted to hospital after ED evaluation had MI. 4% of patients released from EDs after evaluation had MI diagnosed by follow-up cardiac enzymes. An Israeli report showed an 8% ED MI miss rate. Most other studies have found rates of MI after discharge from the ED of less than 5% (1%, 1.7%, 3%, 4%,) and 5.6%. The MI patients released often had non diagnostic cardiograms, atypical histories, and no previous CAD. Unfortunately the missed diagnoses were in younger patients. In a large recent study, Pope evaluated missed AMI sent home from the ED and found that about 5% of patients had ACS, half with MI and half with unstable angina.

Recommendations can be made to avoid releasing ED patients presenting with CP or equivalent symptoms who are at high risk for sudden death. To expedite care, the emergency physician must stratify patients into risk categories:

1. ST-segment elevation
2. NSTE MI or UA
3. Probable Unstable Angina (UA)
4. Possible Unstable Angina
5. Non cardiac disease

All patients in whom acute MI or unstable angina is suspected should be hospitalized. Only those patients who clearly have non cardiac disease should be eliminated from admission for cardiac evaluation.

A standard 12 lead ECG is mandatory in all patients presenting with CP that could possibly be of ACS. An absolutely normal ECG is unusual. Some patients may be discharged once ACS has been excluded from consideration. Most patients with significant underlying cardiac conditions will have an abnormal ECG. A recent prior ECG should be compared for any changes. The patient should be continuously monitored in the ED during the evaluation period with equipment which will record any dysrhythmias or ventricular ectopic activity (VEA). The clinicians must be alert to the presence of any VEA on the monitor since patients with ACS are at higher risk for sudden death from VEA.

All patients on diuretics or who are otherwise at risk for hypokalemia or hypomagnesemia should have these electrolytes measured and abnormalities corrected prior to discharge. Patients with low, moderate or high of ACS, with an abnormal ECG or complex VEA on monitoring need to undergo observation or more definitive evaluation. The shortest, optimum length of time needed for monitoring patients requiring observation is unknown. CP units may answer this and other questions as the science of observation advances.

In spite of widely known risk factors and routine ECG testing, the ED diagnosis of MI
remains elusive in some patients. A review of 100 consecutive autopsies proven MIs revealed a correct diagnosis in only 53%. Unrecognized MIs may be the result of physicians with training deficits. The ECG is the single most important ancillary test for determining whether a patient has sustained an infarction. Unfortunately its lack of sensitivity makes it an inappropriate single tool for screening. The ECG coupled with the patient's history is our standard initial evaluation of patients who may have ACS. The ECG specificity for STEMI is excellent. The ECG can also detect dysrhythmias and ischemia. However, the ECG is often abnormal and nondiagnostic. The ECG can be normal in patients whose infarcts are early or located in "hidden" areas of myocardium.

ECG FACTS

1. 1-6% of ED patients with CP and normal ECG's will be found subsequently to have a MI.
2. 6-21% of patients admitted to a CCU with a normal ECG will have MI.
3. 84% of patients with a STE MI will have a diagnostic ECG in the ED.
4. 56% of patients with NSTE MI will have a diagnostic ECG in the ED.
5. 24% of patients with NSTE MI will have only LVH or LVH with strain on the ECG in the ED.

Patients discharged from ED's who have already sustained a MI are of great concern and the ECG may be helpful in sorting these patients out. Studies have reported that approximately 25% of the missed MIs result from failure to recognize ECG changes and another 25% from failure to admit patients with ECG changes recognized by the physician who then elects to discharge the patient.

Other tests and new approaches hold promise to enhance the Emergency Physician's judgment. Artificial intelligence (AI) applications, new and more rapid enzymes assays, nuclear scans, extended ECGs, and echocardiographic studies have been reported to improve diagnostic accuracy.

Extended Lead ECG

The addition of leads V4R (the right ventricle) and V8, V9 (the posterior wall) to the standard 12 lead will help identify patients who may qualify for thrombolysis. The presence of ST segment elevation in the posterior or RV distribution may not be apparent on the 12 lead ECG.

Twenty Two Lead ECG

This technology measures deviations in myocardial conduction velocity. The ECG is recorded from 22 locations. The signals are filtered, amplified, digitized and quantified beat to beat. The differences between beats are expressed in an ischemia index (a continuous scale from 0-150). Healthy subjects have been reported to have low indexes and patients with ACS high indexes. The 22 lead tracing may have a higher sensitivity with equal specificity over the standard 12 lead ECG for determining which patients had ACS, higher sensitivity with lower specificity for MI, but a lower sensitivity for MI requiring thrombolysis. Full vests with over 100 leads are under development and may more fully map the electrical activity of the heart demonstrating more accuracy. The search for serologic markers of myocardial necrosis has become a mainstay of the clinical diagnosis of MI.

ENZYME ASSAYS

When myocardial cells are damaged, their enzymatic contents leak eventually into the general circulation. Enzyme concentrations measured in venous blood depend on the enzyme's molecular size, its rate of clearance from the blood, and local cardiac lymph and blood flow. In 1954, elevations of aspartate aminotransferase were reported in patients with MI. Since then, many studies have been performed on the contributions which measurements of lactate dehydrogenase (LDH) and creatine phosphokinase (CK) make to the diagnosis of MI. CK has three cytosolic isoenzymes (CK MM, BB, MB) and one mitochondrial isoenzyme of CK (molecular wt of 86,000). CK MM is predominant in both heart and skeletal muscle, CK MB represents 1-30% of total cardiac CK activity and <2% of total skeletal muscle CK activity. One very interesting phenomenon is that the MB percentage of cardiac CK activity will vary with low levels <2% being noted on biopsy specimens taken from normal heart and high levels 25-30% being noted in hearts with chronic LVH and chronic CAD. As CK MB has greater affinity for creatine phosphate than does MM, this increase is thought to be an adaptive response to chronic hypoxia making the transfer of high energy phosphate from ATP to creatine more efficient.

The new immunochemical methods can detect lower levels of CK-MB enzyme. Rapid, serial testing (1 and 3 hours) appears to be more sensitive than single electrophoretic determinations. With newer immunochemical methods lab turnaround times can be reduced or tests can be performed at the bedside. Enzyme values can be made available almost immediately to the emergency physician. Rapid enzymes tests have much lower thresholds for a positive result than older techniques.

In most centers, the ED evaluation of patients with CP includes serum cardiac enzymes. The traditional wisdom banning utilization of these test in the ED, was based on several studies showing that a single determination of CK or CK-MB by electrophoretic technique was not a sensitive screen for MI. There remains a concern that physicians might be misled by false negative enzyme result. Hence, the dictum, "if you order cardiac enzymes, admit the patient!" However, the use of initial enzymes has become virtually universal in most U.S. centers.

One Israeli study suggested a value to ED CK testing as early as 1984; a CK test 4 hours after ED arrival improved the clinicians' diagnostic sensitivity by 34%. More recently studies have shown the potential utility of early and serial enzyme testing in Emergency Department evaluation of patients with CP. These studies have utilized newer, more rapid bedside technology and indicate that panels of enzymes myoglobin, troponin and CK-MB are more sensitive than any single test of combination of two.

Many patients proven to have M.I. have non- diagnostic ECGs. Some patients with non diagnostic ECGs will have positive initial ED enzymes. While some will be false positive, patients with elevated troponins will have higher risk of cardiac events in the hospital. All patients with diagnostic ECGs have subsequently proven MIs, specificity 100%, the sensitivity of ECG alone is low, about 33%.

Rapid serial enzymes testing holds particular promise in identifying patients with MI who have non-diagnostic cardiograms. When CK-MB and other enzymes assays are available, physician judgment concerning patient admission is improved. Since the emergency physician must be concerned about the improper discharge of patients with cardiac disease, the sensitivity of these tests is concerning. The use of a false negative test remains problematic, since few of the studies reported to date have followed patients released from the ED and required enzymatic testing of these patients. While high reported sensitivities reassure some emergency physicians, the practice of most EP unaided by enzyme tests in the ED is 95% sensitive. The sensitivity reported must be balanced against the diligence in finding the missed MIs sent home. Many enzyme study protocols are not designed to find these patients. Unfortunately most studies of enzymatic assays have focused on admitted/observed patients and not had follow up of patients discharged from ED without observation.

The MB CK isoenzyme test for the emergency department is readily available. Test results can return within minutes to the emergency physician or be determined at the bedside. The serial measurement of CK-MB at time of presentation and then 3 hours later in patients with non diagnostic ECGs under observation have a sensitivity of about 85% and specificity of about 95%. It is unlikely that the measurement of CK-MB will achieve the goal of 100% sensitivity. Hence it is important to continue to caution that a single

CK-MB test cannot serve as R/O MI test in the ED.

While CK and CKMB remain the reference diagnostic tests, there are other enzymatic tests available in use.

Subforms Of CKMB

The isoenzymes of CK exist in a single form in tissue. Once released into the serum, these dimeric enzymes interact with plasma carboxypeptidase-which cleaves a terminal lysine from carboxyl terminus of both the M and the B monomer. Subforms of both CK MM and CK MB exist. Use of subform of the MB enzymes demonstrates higher sensitivity than CKMB alone. These subforms of CK isoenzymes can be measured with monoclonal immunoassays directed against each subtype. The normal serum ratios of the CK isoenzyme subforms will vary if there is an increased release rate of the isoenzyme from tissue (such as in MI). With MI, there will be a greater proportion of tissue form present.

Troponin

Is a regulatory protein of the myofibril's contractile apparatus, which is actually a complex of three proteins, troponin C (the calcium binding component), troponin I (the inhibitory component with a molecular wt of 23,000) and troponin T (the tropomyosin component) with a molecular wt of 42,000. Cardiac specific isoforms have been identified for troponin T and troponin I and changes in their concentrations have been investigated for use as an early MI marker. These enzymes are present in very low concentrations in normal sera. In acute cardiac ischemia there seems to be two-phase release- the early rise resulting from transient leakage from a cytosolic pool followed by a delayed but continuous liberation associated with myofilament degradation. Troponin T seems to be the better studied of the two (largely due to earlier development of a specific assay). Both troponin T and I shows an increase within 3 hours of MI and remains evaluated for more than 5 days. Troponin elevations have also been detected in patients with "unstable angina," begging the question of what defines an MI. Troponin may be more sensitive than CKMB. Initial troponin levels have been correlated with patient outcome during hospital stay and at discharge.

Myoglobin

Is a cytoplasmic heme protein has a MW of 17,000, is released earlier than CK from necrotic cells. Detectable serum elevations occur within 1 hour after onset of MI. The peak concentrations occur within 4-12 hours. Serum myoglobin has been correlated with the severity, complications, and prognosis of MI. Admission myoglobin has a sensitivity of 60-70%, with a specificity of 70-90%. Myoglobin is widely distribution within skeletal muscles and serum elevations are caused by muscular injury.

In conclusion, there is no one foolproof enzymatic method available to identify all patients with MI.

Recommendations

1. The ED lab should offer a rapid CKMB, troponin or combined panel of CK, MB, troponin and myoglobin assay, use a mass method reporting ng/ml.
2. A single test or panel that is negative at ED arrival is not a reliable guide to patient disposition. Retain patients for serial serologic and ECG determinations whenever you are considering ACS.
3. Any patient with ECG abnormalities (including LVH). and symptomatic patient with an ECG abnormality should be released without sequential ECG and/or serologic determinations.

Serologic markers may soon be found which reduce the rate of incorrect discharge of ED patients with MI. However, the diagnostic accuracy for patients whose symptoms represent unstable angina, but who have not yet begun to infarct, may not be changed by these tests.

UNSTABLE ANGINA

Is best classified by proximity and severity; Type I: anginal onset within last 3 months without rest pain, Type II: angina at rest within past month, but not within past 48 hours, and Type III: angina at rest within 48 hours.

Unstable angina can also be classified by clinical circumstances; Type A: angina secondary to another clinical condition such as anemia, fever, infection, etc., Type B: angina in absence any complicating condition, and Type C: angina within 2 weeks of documented acute MI.

Troponin has been said to identify some patients with unstable angina. This may be a failure to recognize troponin as a more sensitive marker of cardiac cell damage than CK-MB. Three other areas show promise for evaluating the patient presenting with CP and a non diagnostic ECG, nuclear and echo as well as imaging artificial intelligence.

ARTIFICIAL INTELLIGENCE

Goldman, Baxt and Selker lead the AI efforts with vastly different approaches. Goldman's chest pain algorithm can be applied by clinicians following a patient care plan. Baxt's AI applications involve analyzing multiple data points and constructing nonlinear anagrams for each possible pattern of risk factors. The anagrams are linked to a probability of MI. As many as 60 or more pieces of information can be entered into an anagram, including risk factors, elements of history, findings on exam, and ECG changes. Selker's work embeds an analytic device in the ECG machine and collects a minimal data set, age, gender, and presence or pain. The ECG is interpreted. A probability of MI or ischemia is calculated and displayed on the print out of the ECG. Selker's ACI-TIPI (Acute Coronary Ischemia-Time Insensitive Predictive Instrument) has proven value in selecting patients for the CCU and may have value in selecting patients for discharge home. The physician thus informed makes better selection of patients for CCU admission than the unaided physician. Selker's studies have had excellent patient follow-up and demonstrate the efficacy of a test used in clinical practice. Goldman and Baxt's AI applications have been shown to have a better accuracy in predicting MI than the clinician, but they have not been subjected to effectiveness trials. The result of their clinical use is not known.

NUCLEAR IMAGING SESTAMIBI

The Sestamibi scan has recently been proven to be as safe and accurate as an overnight observation for patients with low to moderate risk chest pain.

ECHOCARDIOGRAPHY

Regional wall motion abnormalities (RWMA) on 2D echo correlate with ischemia and infarction. Regional wall motion abnormalities occur within seconds of coronary occlusion. Immediate echocardiography in the ED could detect RWMA in patients with normal or equivocal ECG'S. ED based reports suggest that a bedside echo is both useful and feasible. Although the problem of inadequate follow-up of discharged patients remains.

The benefits of bedside echo and Sestamibi are a very high sensitivity in absence previous history of CAD and the ability to predict in hospital complications for patients with MI. Information on areas of myocardium remote from region of acute injury which suggests severe coronary stenosis in vessels other than the one which is acute occluded the potential to make other diagnoses such as aortic dissection and pericarditis with effusion.

The use of echo is limited by the availability of trained personnel. The use of Sestamibi is limited by Nuclear Medicine laboratory hours. Neither echocardiography nor nuclear imaging can differentiate acute ischemia from old infarct. Patient with prior CAD and MI require serial enzymatic testing. The echo may not detect transient ischemia unless the ischemic event coincides with the echo examination. However, the Sestamibi scan remains positive up to 3 hours after symptoms have resolved.

Chest pain units offer the possibility of more prolonged and sophisticated evaluation and monitoring. ST segment monitoring may be of value in this setting, detecting silent ischemia or angina. At the present time, careful attention to historical factors will dictate the clinicians' ultimate decision regarding these patients. In the absence of a normal test, ECG, enzymes, echo, or Sestamibi, a suggestive history should prompt further evaluation with observation.

CT SCAN AND MRI

The value of CT and MRI is currently being explored. Their greatest value may be in screening for CAD. Modification of risk factors is a primary care concern and overlaps with the role of the emergency physician in the evaluation of patients presenting with CP. CP patients who can be advised to modify smoking and diet. This advice may have greater impact in the acute setting.

EXERCISE TREADMILL TESTING

In stable patients with risk factors for CAD exercise treadmill testing (ETT) can be undertaken after serial tests are negative or as long as there is low suspicion of an acute event. ETT in patients with undiagnosed CP evaluates the responses of the heart to increased cardiac work. The pattern of response predicts the presence and severity of coronary disease. ECG criteria for an abnormal test include a minimum of 1mm of J point depression, an ST segment that is down sloping, or development of ventricular dysrhythmias. Non ECG criteria of ischemia include failure to achieve a heart rate > 120/minute, a drop in systolic pressure of > 10mmHg at any time during the test, low product of systolic blood pressure x heart rate (< 15,000), or inability to exercise beyond 3 minutes.

Reported sensitivity of ETT for detection of coronary disease varies between 55-70%. Specificities are generally reported to be 80-95% in men and 60-80% in women. The test has been conducted on outpatients and patients have been adequately followed. There is great potential for an ETT in the ED setting. Patients with a history of symptoms consistent with acute ischemia who have a normal ECG and bedside enzyme profile could be tested immediately. Studies on ED patients have demonstrated that an immediate stress test is adequate to rule out acute ischemia in very low risk patients with atypical CP and normal ECG'S.

Recommendation

A provocative stress test for ischemia in a select group of ED patients is useful and underutilized. ETT should be routine in the evaluation of CP after serial tests are negative and in low risk patients with atypical pain.

ROLE OF CHEST PAIN UNITS

The rationale for chest pain units stems from our problems with rapid diagnosis of ACS. There remain several problems with the diagnosis of AMI in the ED. There is a significant and often unknown missed MI rate in the group of patients released from the ED. Many studies of new diagnostic modalities have not followed patients released from the ED. Hence, it is difficult to know if any of these new tests will reduce our misdiagnosis rate. There is an over reliance on existing tests. All patients with CP get an ECG. Many will have a non diagnostic ECG. Abnormal ECGs are a significant challenge to the clinician. Patients with risk factors for CAD and a history suggestive of angina with no evidence of infarction or ischemia, pose another challenge even when the ECG is normal. Patients with underlying heart disease and some risk for sudden death are of concern as well. These patients are plentiful in our EDs and need observation with a rapid, cost effective, comprehensive work up.

Finally, the ED physician interprets data; historical features, ECGs, adjunctive tests with limited accuracy. The use of an initial panel of marker CB, troponin, myoglobin and then serial testing with CK or troponin holds promise for the group of patients with NSTE MI and non diagnostic ECGs. However, these markers will not identify patients with unstable angina. The use of the ACI-TIPI may help address this group since a probability of ACS generated will help sort out this group. The use of a computer interpreted ECG (standard at many centers) may help reduce ECG misinterpretation. Neither ACI-TIPI nor serial CK-MB have been shown to reduce the number of missed MIs released from the ED. Our threshold for admission must remain low enough to capture all patients with ACS. This low threshold for admission and need for serial testing followed by ETT have supported development of CP centers.

ED Chest Pain centers can provide an inexpensive, comfortable, overnight or short stay allowing a more comprehensive evaluation of low risk patients. Data show cost savings with a higher standard of care for these patients in CP centers. Many EDs have established CP Centers or Heart ERs for a variety of reasons, to generate more ED visits, to generate more patients for cardiac evaluation and treatment, to enhance prestige, and to deliver better care to patients with CP and cardiac disease.

Since most of the MIs missed with our current strategy for evaluation of CP could be solved by more prolonged observation, CP Centers or the adoption of ED observation protocols are important adjuncts to care. In a low risk patient, observation with serial enzymes and ECGs for 6, 9, or 12 hours can definitively rule out MI. One of the current foci of research is on finding the shortest protocol, 6 hours. ST segment monitoring may detect ischemia or routine monitoring dysrhythmias. ETT can then safely be offered to further define the presence or absence of CAD after completion of negative serial testing. Sestamibi rest scan followed by stress Sestamibi may allow an alternative to prolonged observation when Sestamibi scan is available. At many different EDs 60-90% of patients with CP or equivalent syndromes, are admitted. Of those that go home 5% have significant ACS, NSTE MI or unstable angina. We have a variety of thresholds for admission.

Recommendations

1. EDs should consider development of CP Centers and specific protocols to enhance CP evaluation.
2. Careful effort should be made to increase the availability of echo Sestamibi scan and ETT for patients in the ED.

REFERENCES

1. Selker HP, Zalenski RJ. An evaluation of technologies for detecting acute cardiac ischemia in the emergency department: a report of the NIH national heart attack alert program. Ann Emerg Med 1997;29:1-87.
2. Pope JH, Ruthazer R, Beshansky JR, et al. Clinical features of emergency department patients presenting with symptoms suggestive of acute cardiac ischemia: a multicenter study. J Thromb Thrombolysis 1998;6:63-74.
3. Braunwald E, Mark DB, Jones RH, et al. Unstable angina: diagnosis and management. In: Clinical Practice Guideline Number 10. Rockville, MD: Agency for Health Care Policy and Research, US Public Health Service, US Department of Health and Human Services, 1994.
4. Fineberg HV, Scadden D, Goldman L. Care of patients with a low probability of acute myocardial infarction:

cost-effectiveness of alternatives to coronary care unit admission. N Engl J Med 1984;310:1301-7.

5. McCarthy BD, Wong JB, Selker HP. Detecting acute cardiac ischemia in the emergency department: a review of the literature. J Gen Intern Med 1990;5:365-73.

6. Lee TH, Rouan GW, Weisberg MC, et al. Clinical characteristics and natural history of patients sent home from the emergency room. Am J Cardiol 1987;60:220-4.

7. McCarthy BD, Beshansky JR, D'Agostino RB, Selker HP. Missed diagnoses of acute myocardial infarction in the emergency department: results from a multicenter study. Ann Emerg Med 1993;22:579-82.

8. Pope JH, Aufderheide TP, Ruthazer R, et al. Missed diagnoses of acute cardiac ischemia in the emergency department. N Engl J Med 2000;342:1163-70.

9. Wackers FJT, Lie KI, Liem KL et al. Potential value of thallium-201 scintigraphy as a means of selecting patients for the coronary care unit. Br Heart J 1979; 41:111-7.

10. Beller GA. Radiopharmaceuticals in nuclear cardiology. In: Beller GA, ed. Clinical Nuclear Cardiology. Philadelphia: Saunders; 1995:37-81.

11. Varetto T, Cantalupi D, Altieri A, et al. Emergency room technetium-99m sestamibi imaging to rule out acute myocardial ischemic events in patients with nondiagnostic electrocardiography. J Am Coll Cardiol 1993; 22:1804-8.

12. Hilton TC, Thompson RC, Williams H, et al. Technetium-99m sestamibi myocardial perfusion imaging in the emergency room evaluation of chest pain. J Am Coll Cardiol 1994;23:1016-22.

13. Tatum JL, Jesse Rl, Kontos MC, et al. Comprehensive strategy for the evaluation and triage of the chest pain patient. Ann Emerg Med 1997;29:116-25.

14. Kontos MC, Jesse RL, Anderson P, et al. Comparison of myocardial perfusion imaging and cardiac troponin I in patients admitted to the emergency department with chest pain. Circulation 1999;99:2073-8.

15. Heller GV, Stowers SA, Hendel RC, et al. Clinical value of acute rest technetium-99m tetrofosmin tomographic myocardial perfusion imaging in patients with acute chest pain and nondiagnostic electrocardiograms. J Am Coll Cardiol 1998;31:1011-7.

16. Weissman IA, Dickinson CZ, Dworkin HJ, O'Neill WW, Juni JE. Cost-effectiveness of myocardial perfusion imaging with SPECT in the emergency department evaluation of patients with unexplained chest pain. Radiology 1996;199:353-7.

17. Radensky PW, Hilton TC, Fulmer H, McLaughlin B, Stowers SA. Potential cost effeectiveness of initial myocardial perfusion imaging for assessment of emergency department patients with chest pain. Am J Cardiol 1997;79: 595-9.

18. Beller GA. Editorial: Acute radionuclide perfusion imaging for evaluation of chest pain in the emergency department: Need for a large clinical trial. J Nucl Cardiol 1996;6:546-9.

19. Jafary F, Udelson JE. Assessment of myocardial perfusion and left ventricular function in acute coronary syndromes: Implications for gated SPECT imaging. In: Germano G, Berman DS eds. Clinical Gated Cardiac SPECT. Futura Publishing, Armonk NY, 1999.

20. Hilton TC, Fulmer H, Abuan T, et al. Ninety-day follow-up of patients in the emergency department with chest pain who undergo initial single-photon emission computed tomographic perfusion scintigraphy with technetium 99m-labeled sestamibi. J Nucl Cardiol 1996;3:308-11.

21. Pozen MW, D'Agostino RB, Selker HP, Sytkowski PA, Hood WB Jr. A predictive instrument to improve coronary care unit admission practices in acute ischemic heart disease: A prospective multicenter clinical trial. N Engl J Med 1984;310:1273-8.

22. Sarasin FP, Reymond JM, Griffith JL, et al. Impact of the acute cardiac ischemia time-insensitive predictive instrument (ACI-TIPI) on the speed of triage decision making for emergency department patients presenting with chest pain: a controlled clinical trial. J Gen Intern Med 1994;9:187-94.

23. Selker HP, Beshansky JR, Griffith JL, et al. Use of the acute cardiac time-insensitive predictive instrument (ACI-TIPI) to assist with triage of patients with chest pain or other symptoms suggestive of acute cardiac ischemia: a multicenter, controlled clinical trial. Ann Intern Med 1998;129:845-55.

24. Lee TH, Pearson DS, Johnson PA, et al. Failure of information as an intervention to modify clinical management: A time-series trial in patients with acute chest pain. Ann Intern Med 1995;122:434-7.

25. Roberts RR, Zalenski RJ, Mensah EK, et al. Costs of an emergency department-based accelerated diagnostic protocol vs. hospitalization in patients with chest pain: a randomized controlled trial. JAMA 1997;278:1670-6.

26. Farkouh ME, Smars P, Reeder GS, et al. A clinical trial of a chest pain observation unit for patients with unstable angina. N Engl J Med 1998;339:1882-8.

27. Duca MD, Giri S, Wu AHB, et al. Comparison of acute rest myocardial perfusion imaging and serum markers of myocardial injury in patients with chest pain syndromes. J Nucl Cardiol 1999;6:570-6.

28. Adams JE III, Bodor GS, Davila-Roman VG, et al. Cardiac troponin I: a marker with high specificity for cardiac injury. Circulation 1993;88:101-6.

29. Zimmerman J, Fromm R, Meyer D, et al. Diagnostic marker cooperative study for the diagnosis of

myocardial infarction. Circulation 1999;99:1671-7.
30. Newby LK, Christenson RH, Ohman EM, et al. Value of serial troponin T measures for early and late risk
    stratification in patients with acute coronary syndromes. Circulation1998;98:1853-9

THE NEW 2000 ACLS GUIDELINES

Walter N. Simmons, M.D., M.P.H & David Brodkin*

Cardiovascular disease accounts for approximately one half of the 2 million deaths in the U. S each year. Of the deaths related to cardiovascular disease, 350,000 people die before reaching the hospital. The population is aging, and with it the incidence of cardiac arrests will increase because the prevalence of heart disease and arrhythmias increases with advancing age. With this in mind, the American Heart Association (AHA), the Committee on Emergency Cardiovascular Care, and the Subcommittees on Basic Life Support, Advanced Cardiac Life Support, and Pediatric Resuscitation's have developed cardiopulmonary resuscitation (CPR) and emergency cardiac care (ECC) guidelines for both the adult and for the pediatric population.

The AHA guidelines began to take shape after Kouwenhoven et. al became one of the first groups to present positive patient outcomes in closed-chest (CPR) at Johns Hopkins University in 1960. At that time Kowenhoven's group reported a 70% survival-to-discharge rate in patients ranging in age from 2 months to 80 years. To date these results have never been replicated. These results, however, were sufficient to create a movement to determine standardized treatments for those individuals suffering from life-threatening cardiac events. In this effort, the first standardized CPR guidelines were published by the AHA in 1974 and have since been updated in 1980, 1986, 1992 and the latest version in 2000.

The 2000 AHA guidelines have been renovated to include the growing body of evidence supporting the different methods of CPR and the use of various medications used in resuscitation. The 2000 guidelines are the first to have extensive international participation in their development with at least 50% of participants involved in development residing outside the United States. The new guidelines are generally considered to be more evidence-based then previous versions. To this end, a new classification system has been instilled into the 2000 guidelines as a graded representation of the AHA panel's view of the strength of their recommendation. The classifications are based upon the level of supporting evidence. Class I recommendations

---

* Walter N. Simmons, M.D., M.P.H., Fellow in Emergency Medicine, Brown University/Rhode Island Hospital
David Brodkin, University of Massachusetts School of Medicine, Worchester, Mass.

are defined as those with proven efficacy. Class IIa are acceptable and believed to be useful but not completely proven. Class IIb are clearly unproven but thought to be helpful. Class intermediate states that there is not enough evidence for the AHA's recommendation. Lastly, class IIı are defined as completely unacceptable.

With evidence-based guidelines in place, the question of which patients are most likely to survive CPR can be asked. To answer this question, Bedell et. al studied a population with a high chance of needing CPR, home-bound individuals. Bedell described home-bound patients as those persons who had not pursued activities outside the home before their acute illness. This definition proves to be an important marker for the outcome of CPR. In Bedell's study, only 4% of homebound patients survived as compared with 27% of non-homebound patients. In addition, several studies have shown that patients without response in the field to CPR had no successful discharges to home from the hospital. This was consistent with the pediatric population. Resuscitations on the medical wards and in the intensive care units (ICU) have lower success rates than in specialized areas such as the cardiac care unit, operating room, or emergency department. Low success rates on the medical wards most likely reflects a delay in detection, while the low rates of successful resuscitation in the ICUs is probably the result of illness severity in the ICU patient population.

The survival-to-discharge rate after CPR taken from numerous studies varies from 0% to 29%, and age was or was not a factor depending on the study. Several consistencies can have been discovered from large post-hoc analysis. An arrhythmia amenable to defibrillation is an important characteristic in terms of a successful CPR. In general, individuals have improved outcomes if the initial rhythm upon initiation of CPR is ventricular fibrillation (VF) or ventricular tachycardia (VT). When analyzed separately, the elderly who do present with VT or VF appear to have similar resuscitation success rates as seen in younger adults. Success is defined as the return of spontaneous circulation (ROSC) following CPR. A pulse correlates with a higher discharge rate from the hospital. Another important factor contributing to surviving CPR is the duration of the arrest. It also appears that, in the elderly, the level of fitness and activity level before CPR relates to higher rates of successful CPR.

CPR, as recommended by the American Heart Association, begins with activating the emergency response system and performing a primary ABCD Survey. The A represents assessing and opening the airway. B is to check for breathing and if absent to provide positive-pressure ventilations. C is to appreciate circulation and give chest compressions if necessary. D is for defibrillation, if after assessment, the patient is found to be in VF or pulseless VT. If responsiveness is decreased or absent a defibrillator should be immediately requested and then the ABCD survey should begin. Although the order of the survey is generally accepted, much of the rest of the way in which the ABCD survey is conducted is under debate. This discussion is primarily concerned with mechanical and bystander ventilation. It has been argued that to put an endotracheal (ET) tube into the oropharynx is time consuming and the use of a bag-valve mask can greatly insufflate the stomach. The placement of an ET tube afterward positive ventilation can stimulate the posterior pharynx and result in the patient vomiting and aspirating. Additionally, even skilled intubators take approximately 30-40 seconds to place an ET tube. It has been suggested that during this time, chest compressions are generally halted to allow for an easier intubation. The 30 seconds without chest compression and cerebral blood flow may translate into increasing morbidity. To provide evidence for this argument, a study conducted in Seattle, Washington demonstrated that chest compression alone improved survival in telephone CPR. Future studies are needed to help end this debate.

The determination of pulse has also been examined recently with interesting results. Multiple studies have found that physicians and the lay person to be very poor at determining peripheral pulses. For the lay person, it was no better than approximately 50%, and the odds were not much improved for most physicians. It is now recommended by the AHA that lay persons should not perform pulse checks but should instead look for signs of breathing and chest movement. If no breathing or movement is present, then it is appropriate to proceed with CPR. For the physician, the decision of which pulse to test remains. Elderly patients have a high likelihood of having carotid plaques, with the average being two plaques and a large percentage possessing more than three carotid plaques. This makes palpation of the carotid artery a dangerous proposition. Palpation at the carotid artery may increase risk for either occluding carotid flow or disrupting a plaque thus causing distal embolization. A lack of pulsation in the carotid artery may, therefore, not indicate lack of circulation. A possible alternative would be to use the femoral pulse as a measure of circulation.

Circulatory management during a cardiac arrest includes cardiac chest compressions. Compressions are reported to achieve 25-30% of the normal cardiac output. Two theories predominate for how chest compressions achieve this result. The cardiac pump theory suggests that the heart is compressed between the sternum and the spine and that this results in blood being squeezed into the systemic and pulmonary circulation. A more recent theory, the thoracic pump model, suggests that pressure changes in the thorax are responsible for forward blood flow and the heart is merely a conduit. There are several new devices reported to increase cardiac output. The most promising appears to be the active compression-decompression device (ACD), although little hard evidence exists to support the recommendation of its use. According to the new AHA guidelines, 100 beats per minute (bpm) is recommended to the old recommendation of 80 bpm.

After the ABCD survey--including defibrillation--the AHA recommends the use of certain medications. Many new drugs have been added to the treatment algorithms and there have been some dramatic changes to the recommended medications. The use of antiarrythmics has undergone significant changes from the prior iterations of the guidelines. The AHA now states that antiarrhythmic medications should be considered for patients in VT/VF who have not converted after three defibrillation attempts and administration of a vasopressor. While there are multiple antiarrhythmics available to physicians, the guidelines state that only one should be used. If that antiarrhythmic does not work, then electrical cardioversion should be again be attempted. Amiodarone is one of the medications that was added to the VT/VF algorithm. It has replaced lidocaine as a first-line antiarrhythmic, and is now recommended for use during the management of VT/VF. Amiodarone is a class III antidysrhythmic (potassium channel blocker) with some additional class I (sodium channel blocking), class II (beta adrenergic blocking), and class IV (calcium channel blocking) effects. It is given a Class IIb by the AHA in terms of its proven effectiveness.

Some of the evidence supporting amiodarone comes from Kudenchuk who studied its use in out-of-hospital cardiac arrest due to VF. In this study, there were 504 patients with cardiac arrest in VF or pulseless VT who had received ≥ 3 shocks, were intubated, and were given 1mg epinephrine IV. The participants were randomized to 300 mg amiodarone IV or placebo. He found that amiodarone-treated patients were more likely to survive the hospital admission with spontaneous circulation than placebo patients (44% vs. 34%). However, there was no significant difference in terms of survival to hospital discharge (13.4% vs. 13.2%) or good neurological outcome (7.3% vs. 6.6%). Another study adding to the evidence that Amiodorone is a good choice in some patients comes from the recently completed ALIVE study. The ALIVE study investigated out-of-hospital cardiac arrest due to VF and was a manufacturer-supported Canadian pre-hospital trial of comparing amiodarone to lidocaine. Preliminary results were announced at the North American Society of Pacing and Electrophysiology in March 2001. The results indicate that amiodarone use was associated with improved ROSC and survival to hospital admission compared to lidocaine. The ALIVE study does, however, state that "the use of amiodarone in refractory pulseless VT/VF should not be considered the current 'standard of care' for this condition" and that "until ongoing or future research clarifies this issue, emergency physicians should use their own discretion regarding anti-arrhythmic therapy in patients with cardiac arrest." The current IV dosing of amiodarone for ventricular tachyarrhythmias begins with rapid infusion of 150mg over 10 minutes. That is followed by slow infusion of 360mg over 6 hours (1mg/min). Maintenance infusion then continues at 0.5mg/min. Any infusion greater than 2 hours requires a glass bottle.

Lidocaine may be used to treat VT as well, though there is no evidence that it improves outcomes. 17 It is given a class indeterminate recommendation in the 2000 AHA Guidelines. Multiple studies have demonstrated that lidocaine is successful in converting VT to sinus rhythm in only 20–30% of cases. It still clearly has a place in the treatment of patients with stable VT. Advantages of lidocaine include ease of dosing and administration (which allow it to be administered more rapidly than procainamide or amiodarone), rapid effect (when it does work), minimal side effect profile, and low cost. Physicians that choose to use lidocaine must be prepared to move on to second-line medications rapidly in cases when lidocaine is ineffective. Procainamide and amiodarone, on the other hand, are far more successful at converting VT.

Another major addition to the AHA algorithms is the use of vasopressin as an alternative vasopressor agent to epinephrine. The posterior pituitary gland releases vasopressin as a peptide hormone. Vasopressin is normally released in response to hypovolemia and hypotension major hemorrhage, severe stress, or head injury or increased plasma osmolality. Vasopressin receptors have been divided into V_1 and V_2 receptor subtypes. The V_1 subtype appears to be predominately responsible for blood pressure control, causing vasoconstriction when activated. Because of its strong vasopressive effects and low toxicity, it has the opportunity to become the primary drug for the management of VT/VF. This would suggest vasopressin is a better drug than epinephrine. Vasopressin receives a Class IIb recommendation, as does epinephrine. It should be used only once as its effect is prolonged (40 minutes). Epinephrine had previously been considered the sole first line vasopressor agent used in VT/VF. Epinephrine acts strongly on the α1 and α2 receptors which act on the heart and contract peripheral arteries. They, therefore, increase systemic vascular resistance and allow blood to preferentially shunt to the brain and coronary arteries. However, their beta agonist effects increase myocardial oxygen requirement and may cause islands of ischemic injury. The results may be better if esmolol is added to block epinephrine's beta properties.

Two major studies compare the use of vasopressin and epinephrine. The first was conducted in 1997 when Lindner et al published the first randomized, double-blind trial of vasopressin vs. epinephrine. In this pre-hospital study, 40 VF patients that were resistant to initial CPR and defibrillation were randomized to receive either epinephrine 1 mg or vasopressin 40 units. Further standard AHA recommended measures were then taken. Vasopressin was associated with statistically significant improvements in ROSC (16/20 patients vs. 11/20 patients) and survival to hospital admission (14/20 patients vs. 7/20 patients). Survivors to hospital discharge included 8/20 patients in the vasopressin group vs. 3/20 patients in the epinephrine group. However, the difference between vasopressin and epinephrine in this group was not statistically significant because of the small study size.

A second larger study published in July 2001 by Stiell et al showed no benefit of vasopressin vs. epinephrine. Two hundred patients were randomized to receive either a single dose of vasopressin 40 units or epinephrine 1 mg. Patients in either group that failed to respond after the first dose received subsequent doses of epinephrine (1 mg every 3-5 minutes). The results of the study showed no difference between the two groups in ROSC, survival to hospital discharge, or neurological outcome. The authors concluded that they "cannot recommend the routine use of vasopressin for in-hospital cardiac arrest patients, and disagree with American Heart Association guidelines". Based on these studies, vasopressin is now considered an alternative to epinephrine in its use for VT/VF.

Epinephrine does, however, remain the first line medication for management of pulseless electrical activity (PEA) and asystole. The use of high-dose epinephrine has been extensively investigated in multiple large animal studies. Epinephrine in these doses has been shown to decrease cardiac contractility after resuscitation. Two studies conducted by C. Brown showed there to be no benefit to high-dose epinephrine, with an associated increased amount of premature ventricular beats, increased incidence of ventricular fibrillation, and an increased amount of energy needed to defibrillate. Post-resuscitation survival was decreased. 20 Because of these and other studies, the use of high dose epinephrine receives a recommendation of Class Indeterminate by the AHA.

For new drug development for cardiopulmonary resuscitation the selective α2 agonists may be a step in the right direction. An alternative vasopressor agent, α-methylnorepinephrine, has been investigated. It has been shown to result in a better cardiac output while not increasing the oxygen demand. It was thought to be as effective as epinephrine for initial cardiac resuscitation but to provide better post-resuscitation myocardial function and survival.

Other drugs used during CPR include magnesium, procainamide, and sotalol. Magnesium may be indicated in patients with torsades de pointes or hypomagnesia. It is a Class IIb recommendation. Procainamide is a Class IIb recommendation for intermittent or recurrent VF/VT. Due to its long infusion time, there is not much evidence regarding its use during CPR. Sotalol is a second line option in the treatment of stable ventricular tachycardia. If used prophylactic ally, it may cause torsades de pointes and increase mortality. Bretylium is no longer a part of the ACLS algorithm due to an unavailability of raw materials to produce the drug.

The 2000 AHA Guidelines also present changes for the use of defibrillation during resuscitation. It recognizes that the in-hospital survival is heavily reliant on the actions occurring before patients arrive at the hospital. Specifically, defibrillating patients early is a key component of the protocol. Though there is not much definitive evidence, the guideline experts endorsed the concept that cardiac arrest victims should be evaluated, treated, and defibrillated for VF within a short interval of time from collapse to arrest. The problem in both the in-hospital and out-of-hospital settings has been how to best achieve early defibrillation. The concept of a centralized response in which all advanced life support tools are frantically pushed in a single "code 911 cart" cannot possibly be achieved. This leads to the idea of strategically placing automated external defibrillators (AED's) within a hospital and associated outpatient clinics. It is felt that these AED's could facilitate much earlier defibrillation if a larger number are available and if a greater range of healthcare personnel were authorized to operate them. One example of an AHA goal objective is the achievement an interval from collapse to first shock of less than 3 minutes in greater than 90% of arrests (for in-hospital and ambulatory care areas). While this is an example of a specific performance goal, this is not an official AHA recommendation. Despite the lack of hard evidence, it is clear that better outcomes may be achieved if all ACLS providers are trained in CPR and AED defibrillation.

Since the release of the 1992 version of the AHA Guidelines, much evidence on the efficacy of the various components of the algorithm have been compiled. This evidence was systematically evaluated and incorporated into the 2000 version, thus creating a guideline which is substantially improved over the previous version. This evaluation also allowed the guideline to classify the various AHA panel recommendations. Investigators continue to search for more effective methods and means of resuscitation; thus, the AHA guidelines continue to be a work-in-process. There are on-going conferences to update and improve the next version of the guidelines, which is purported to be more evidence-based. At the time of this writing a firm date has not been set for the next version's publication.

REFERENCES

1. Hennekens CH: Update on aspirin in the treatment and prevention of cardiovascular disease. *Am Heart J*, 1999 Apr; 137(4 Pt 2): S9-S13.
2. Eaton CB, Anthony D: Cardiovascular disease and the maturing woman. *Clinics in Family Practice*, 2002 Mar; 4(1); 71-88.
3. Liu LL, Carlisle AS: Management of cardiopulmonary resuscitation. *Anesthesiol Clin North America*, 2000 Mar; 18(1): 143-58, vii

4. Kudenchuk PJ: Advanced cardiac life support antiarrhythmic drugs. *Cardiol Clin*, 2002 Feb; 20(1); 79-87.
5. American Heart Association, International Liaison Committee on Resuscitation: Guidelines 2000 for cardiopulmonary resuscitation and emergency cardiovascular care. *Circulation*, 2000, 102(suppl I).
6. Thel MC, O'Connor CM: Cardiopulmonary resuscitation: historical perspective to recent investigations. *Am Heart J*, 1999 Jan; 137(1): 39-48.
7. Manning JE; Katz LM: Cardiopulmonary and cerebral resuscitation. *Crit Care Clin*. 2000 Oct; 16(4): 659 -79.
8. De Maio VJ, Stiell IG, Spaite DW, et al: CPR-only survivors of out-of-hospital cardiac arrest: implications for out-of-hospital care and cardiac arrest research methodology. *Ann Emerg Med*. 2001 Jun; 37(6): 602-8.
9. Ip SP, Leung YF, Ip CY, et al: Outcomes of critically ill elderly patients: is high-dependency care for geriatric patients worthwhile? *Crit Care Med*. 1999 Nov; 27(11): 2351-7.
10. Katz SH; Falk JL: Misplaced endotracheal tubes by paramedics in an urban emergency medical services system. *Ann Emerg Med*, 2001, Jan; 37(1): 32-7.
11. Cobb LA, Fahrenbruch CE, Walsh TR, et al: Influence of cardiopulmonary resuscitation prior to defibrillation in patients with out-of-hospital ventricular fibrillation. *JAMA*. 1999; 281:1182-1188.
12. Otto CW: Cardiac arrest and monitoring. *Anesthesiol Clin North America*, 2001 Dec; 19(4): 717-26, viii.
13. Wein TH, Bornstein NM: Stroke prevention: cardiac and carotid-related stroke. *Neurol Clin*, 2000 May; 18(2): 321-41.
14. Podrazik PM, Schwartz JB: Cardiovascular pharmacology of aging. *Cardiol Clin*, 1999 Feb; 17(1): 17-34.
15. Atkins DL, Dorian P, Gonzalez ER, et al: Treatment of tachyarrhythmias. *Ann Emerg Med*, 2001 Apr; 37(4 Suppl): S91-109.
16. Voelckel WG, Lurie KG, McKnite S, et al: Effects of epinephrine and vasopressin in a piglet model of prolonged ventricular fibrillation and cardiopulmonary resuscitation. *Crit Care Med*, 2002 May; 30(5): 957-62.
17. Wenzel V, Lindner KH: Arginine vasopressin during cardiopulmonary resuscitation: laboratory evidence. clinical experience and recommendations, and a view to the future. *Crit Care Med*, 2002 Apr; 30(4 Suppl): S157-61.
18. Wessel DL: Managing low cardiac output syndrome after congenital heart surgery. *Crit Care Med*, 2001 Oct; 29(10 Suppl): S220-30.
19. Stiell IG, Hébert PC, Wells GA, et al: Vasopressin versus epinephrine for inhospital cardiac arrest: a randomised controlled trial. *Lancet*, 2001 Jul; 358(9276): 105-9.
20. Brown C, Wiklund L, Bar-Joseph G, et al: Future directions for resuscitation research. IV. Innovative advanced life support pharmacology. *Resuscitation*, 1996 Dec; 33(2): 163-77.
21. Sun S, Weil MH, Tang W, et al: alpha-Methylnorepinephrine, a selective alpha2-adrenergic agonist for cardiac resuscitation. *J Am Coll Cardiol*, Mar 2001; 37(3): 951-6.
22. Cummins RO, White RD, Pepe PE: Ventricular fibrillation, automatic external defibrillators, and the United States Food and Drug Administration: confrontation without comprehension. *Ann Emerg Med*, 1995 Nov; 26(5): 621-31; discussion 632-4.

ATLS UPDATE: CASE STUDIES IN TRAUMA

Daren Girard, M.D. [*]

OVERVIEW

Trauma is the leading cause of death in the first four decades of life and the third leading of all causes of mortality. Furthermore, for every person killed, three others are permanently disabled. Annual trauma-related costs in the United States are in excess of $400 billion. Advanced Trauma Life Support (ATLS) is a model of trauma care endorsed by the American College of Surgeons Committee on Trauma. The first courses were conducted in 1980 with the goal of disseminating a "safe, reliable method for the immediate management of the injured patient." The latest edition of this document, the sixth, was released in 1997. The seventh edition is expected in June 2002. International ATLS programs began in 1987. Currently, 29 countries are authorized to provide ATLS training. More than 225,000 doctors have been certified worldwide.

CASE ONE

History

A 22 year-old male was the unrestrained driver in a road traffic accident (RTA) when his vehicle collided head-on with St. James's Gate. A strong odor of alcohol exudes from the patient. He has an obvious large scalp laceration and is combative. His Glasgow Coma Score (GCS) is 10. The patient's vital signs are HR 105, BP 110/75, RR 24.

Initial Management

---

[*] Daren Girard, M.D., Assistant Professor of Medicine at Brown University, Department of Emergency Medicine, The Miriam Hospital, Providence, Rhode Island

During transport to the emergency department (ED), emergency medical staff (EMS) initiate resuscitation efforts: The patient is placed in a cervical collar and full spinal immobilization. He is provided with high-flow supplemental oxygen. Two large-bore intravenous lines are secured.

Primary Survey

On arrival to the ED, emergency staff triage the patient immediately to the resuscitation area. The patient promptly begins to vomit.

Airway

An awake and alert patient with normal voice quality who answers questions appropriately has no immediate airway problem. Still, regardless of the results of the initial airway evaluation, all trauma patients require regular reassessment of their airway status. This patient's airway is in jeopardy. He has evidence of head injury, a GCS of 10, and is vomiting. His airway needs to be protected with a cuffed endotracheal tube (ETT) secured in the trachea. Intubating this patient will decrease the chance of contaminating his lung with vomit, blood, and secretions. This is important because aspiration and contamination of the airways could complicate his recovery. The first step in protecting this patient's airway is to logroll him onto his side, maintaining full spinal immobilization. Spinal precautions are essential because 1% of all trauma patients have a cervical spine injury. This figure increases to 5% in those with head-injury and 8% in those with a GCS of 8 or less. Next, the patient should be intubated using the rapid sequence technique.

Indications For Definitive Airway in Trauma

Besides apnea, ventilatory failure, and refractory hypoxia, other indications for a definitive airway in trauma are as follows:

1. Massive facial injury
2. Head injury with GCS < 8
3. Multiple trauma with persistent hypotension
4. Thermal injury to the airway
5. Penetrating injury to the neck (zones II or III)
6. Blunt injury to the neck with expanding hematoma or voice change

Rapid Sequence Intubation (RSI)

Rapid sequence intubation employs the use of neuromuscular blockade and sedative-hypnotics to facilitate intubation. The contraindications for RSI are if the oropharynx is obstructed so that the jaw cannot be opened or if the patient cannot be ventilated using a bag-valve mask (BVM). Rapid sequence intubation requires attention to the six Ps.

1. Planning
2. Pre-oxygenation

3. Pre-medication
4. Paralytics
5. Placement of ETT
6. Post-procedure management

Planning

A surgical airway may be necessary if the patient cannot be intubated. Preparations should be made for this possibility.

Pre-oxygenation

In the spontaneously breathing patient, adequate pre-oxygenation is accomplished by a few minutes of 100% oxygen by facemask. This removes nitrogen from the lungs and creates a reservoir of pure oxygen helping the patient to better tolerate a brief period of apnea during the intubation process. The patient with minimal respiratory efforts requires BVM ventilation with the application of cricoid pressure, Sellick's maneuver.

Pre-medication

Children less than 6 years old, require atropine to blunt the vagal response to laryngoscopy. The dose is 0.02 mg/kg with a minimum dose of 0.1 mg and a maximum of 0.5 mg. In head injured patients, lidocaine is recommended to limit the increases in intra-cranial pressure that may accompany intubation. The dose is 1.5 mg/kg.

Paralytics

Etomidate is a GABA agonist that does not increase intra-cranial pressure, nor does it have significant cardiovascular depressant effects. Because trauma patients are typically volume depleted and have a high risk of head injury, etomidate 0.3 mg/kg is commonly used as an induction agent in this setting. If neither of these conditions is suspected, thiopental in doses of 2-3 mg/kg is appropriate for induction. Rocuronium is a non-depolarizing neuromuscular blocking agent given in doses of 0.9 mg/kg. It is also reported to attenuate increases in intra-cranial pressure and is the preferred paralytic for use in patients with head injuries.   Otherwise, 1.5 mg/kg of succinlycholine is appropriated for paralysis.

Placement

Maintaining cervical spine immobilization is essential.   This is a three-person procedure with one person ensuring in-line immobilization, another performing Sellick's maneuver, and the third intubating the patient.

Post-procedure

Endotracheal tube placement should be confirmed using a variety of techniques. The most important of these is the operator's direct observation of the tube passing through the vocal cords. Other measures include observation of chest expansion, auscultation of the chest and abdomen, and detection of end-tidal carbon dioxide. A post-intubation chest X-ray (CXR) should be reviewed. The patient will also require ongoing sedation and paralysis with standard agents.

CASE TWO

History

A 32 year-old male was struck repeatedly about the chest and back with a hurly. He is awake, alert, and talking with a GCS=14. His vital signs are HR 105, BP 110/75, RR 30.

Primary Survey

The patient is awake and answers questions appropriately with a normal voice. He is complaining of right-sided chest pain and states, "I can't breathe".

Breathing

The patient becomes increasingly anxious, tachypneic, and tachycardic. His oxygen saturation drops to 85% on the monitor. His trachea becomes deviated and the breath sounds are decreased on the right side. The latest systolic blood pressure measurement is 85 mm Hg.

Tension Pneumothorax

Tension pneumothorax must be identified early in the primary survey. The physical exam findings include unilateral absence of breath sounds, tracheal deviation, and hypotension. The treatment is immediate needle decompression followed by tube thoracostomy.

CASE THREE

History

A 42 year-old female was unrestrained in an RTA and was ejected from her vehicle. She has a diminished level of consciousness. She is confused and moaning with a GCS of 11. Her vital signs are HR 120, BP 85/45, RR 25.

Primary Survey

The patient is brought to the ED unconscious. She is intubated because of a strong suspicion of head injury, low GCS, and hypotension. After intubation, breath sounds are clear, bilaterally, and symmetric.

Circulation

This patient is hypotensive in the setting of significant blunt trauma. There are a variety of etiologies for shock, but the most likely cause in the trauma patient is hypovolemia from acute blood loss. Tension pneumothorax and pericardial tamponade can also cause hypotension. The latter is more common after penetrating injuries to the chest. In the adult trauma patient, isolated intra-cranial bleeding patient does not cause significant hypotension. Accordingly, occult blood loss should be suspected in the head-injured patient with low blood pressure. Intra-abdominal hemorrhage is the most common source of occult blood loss in these patients. Hemothorax, bleeding as a result of long bone and pelvic fractures, and obvious external bleeding from lacerations can each be sufficient to produce hypotension.

FAST Ultrasound

The FAST scan stands for focused abdominal sonography in trauma. This technology is portable and can be rapidly obtained at the bedside of a critically-injured patient at the same time other members of the trauma team direct the resuscitative efforts and perform procedures. Numerous large studies have shown that non-radiologists, emergency physicians and surgeons, can interpret these scans with a high degree of sensitivity and thereby make important decisions regarding the next steps in the patient's care. A typical decision algorithm now in place at many U.S. trauma centers is as follows:

1. An unstable patient with a positive FAST scan will have an exploratory laparotomy
2. A stable patient with a positive FAST scan will have a CT scan of the abdomen and pelvis to better clarify the injury
3. An unstable patient with a negative FAST scan will undergo further testing to delineate the cause of shock, for example DPL, chest X-ray, etc.
4. A stable patient with a negative FAST scan can be observed

CASE FOUR

History

A young male is involved in an RTA. He veered off Strand Road into a brick wall in a single-car accident that minimally damaged his vehicle. The patient is unconscious with a GCS of three. His vital signs are HR 100 BP, 105/75, RR 10.

Primary Survey

The patient arrives to the ED unconscious. The team prepares to intubate. His breath sounds are clear and symmetric, but with minimal respiratory efforts. His peripheral pulses are full. The team finds no obvious external evidence of trauma and the patient's pupils are 3 mm bilaterally and sluggishly reactive.

Disability

In the ABCDE scheme of trauma care, "D" stands for disability. This underscores the importance of a careful neurological exam during the secondary survey. It also stands for dextrose and drugs, both of which complicate the management of the unresponsive trauma victim. Hypoglycemia and drug intoxications can result in altered mental status. Many times, these conditions are pre-existing and are, in fact, the cause of the accident. Patients with no obvious injuries but severely depressed mental status should receive naloxone as well as a bedside glucose determination before intubation.

CASE FIVE

History

An older man is found down on Bachelor's Quay alongside several empty pints of Guinness. The patient has a decreased level of consciousness with incomprehensible speech. His GCS is 12. with vital signs of HR 100 BP, 105/70, RR 20.

Primary Survey

The patient is presently protecting a patent airway. He has clear breath sounds bilaterally. His pulses are full and equal.

Exposure

The patient's clothing is removed and he is examined from head-to-toe. He is log rolled with full spinal protection. A 0.8 cm stab wound is noted on his left flank. A detailed secondary survey includes a complete physical examination. Especially in patients with diminished responsiveness and ethanol intoxication. Rigorous attention to detail may provide the only clue to a potentially serious injury. Hemotympanum may be the only finding to suggest basilar skull fracture. Inspection of the back, axillae, and perineum may reveal important penetrating injuries that are not otherwise apparent.

Penetrating Flank Injury

Historically, patients with this type of injury underwent mandatory surgical exploration. Now, a combination of serial physical examination, triple-contrast CT, and DPL, have minimized the number of operations performed. Triple-contrast CT (oral, intravenous, and rectal) has a sensitivity of 89-100%, and specificity of 98-100%. With this more selective approach, few injuries are missed while a greater number of patients are spared exploratory laparotomy and its attendant complications.

CASE SIX

History

A 42 year-old male was unrestrained in a RTA. He ran a light and struck a coach of American tourists on Leeson Street. He is alert and talking with a GCS of 15. His vital signs are HR 110, BP 120/75, RR 20.

Primary Survey

The patient has a patent airway. His breath sounds are clear bilaterally. He has full peripheral pulses.

Secondary Survey

A detailed physical exam is completed. The only finding is an anterior chest wall contusion. CXR is obtained.

Traumatic Aortic Injury

The majority of patients with this injury die at the scene of the accident. This injury occurs when rapid deceleration forces are transmitted to the chest wall, as occurs in a high-speed RTA or a fall from a significant height. Patients who survive to the ED have a mortality rate that is directly related to the delay in diagnosis, making rapid diagnosis of this condition a potentially life-saving endeavor. Chest Xray findings suggestive of traumatic aortic injury are as follows:

1. First and second rib fractures
2. Obscuration of the aortic knob
3. Deviation of the trachea to the right
4. Pleural cap
5. Depression of the left main stem bronchus
6. Obliteration of the aorto-pulmonary window
7. Deviation of the naso-gastric tube to the right

Contrast Enhanced Spiral CT

New generation spiral CT scanners are now available. Many large studies have evaluated the use of these newer machines in the diagnosis of traumatic aortic injury and have repeatedly demonstrated a sensitivity of 99.8-100%. This corresponds to a negative predictive value of a negative scan of 100%. In other words, this devastating injury can be reliably ruled-out if the CT scan is negative.

REFERENCES

ATLS Manual 6th Edition 1997, Published by the American College of Surgeons, Chicago

PEDIATRIC TRAUMA

Scott J. Cohen, M.D. *

(Adapted from A.P.L.S. Pediatric Emergency Medicine Course, and Harriet Lane Pediatric Handbook)

CHILDREN ARE DIFFERENT

- Smaller body size
- Greater relative body surface area
- Internal organs are more anterior and protected by less subcutaneous fat
- Differences in pediatric airway; Greater airway resistance and smaller, more anterior airway makes airway management more difficult and higher likely need for intubation
- Head-to-body ratio greater making associated head injury more common
- Presence of physes -- Salter-Harris fractures
- Body size allows for greater distribution of forces; therefore children are more likely to suffer injuries resulting in multiple trauma
- Children's blood pressure may be maintained with up to 30% acute blood loss; they compensate with increased heart rate and systemic vascular resistance; after 30% loss however, their blood pressure drops precipitously

MANAGEMENT

Airway

- Open airway using jaw thrust maneuver and maintain spinal precautions as needed

---

* Scott J. Cohen, M.D., Director, Global Pediatric Alliance, Oakland, California

- Immobilize cervical spine with semirigid collar
- If airway is not maintainable, institute rapid sequence induction and endotracheal intubation
- Suction blood, secretion, and vomitus from mouth; inspect mouth for foreign body and broken teeth
- Consider oral airway in an unconscious child who has spontaneous respirations

Breathing

- Administer bag-valve-mask ventilation for patients who do not have spontaneous and effective respirations
- Indications for intubation:
    apnea,
    hypoventilation,
    hypoxemia/cyanosis,
    flail chest,
    comatose or rapidly declining mental status
    shock unresponsive to volume resuscitation
- Evaluate for signs of tension pneumothorax:
    Poor perfusion
    Severe respiratory distress
    Distended neck veins
    Tracheal deviation
    Asymmetric or absent breath sounds on side of injury
- If pneumothorax suspected, a needle thoracostomy should be performed, followed by placement of chest tube

Circulation

- Apply direct pressure to external bleeding
- Look for signs of shock:
    Tachycardia
    Decreased mental status
    Cool extremities
    Narrowed pulse pressure
    Poor peripheral perfusion
- Administer 20cc/kg normal saline IV/IO for any signs of volume loss; repeat as needed
- Administer 10-15cc/kg packed RBC's if patient hypotensive, or if remains in shock after 2 boluses of normal saline at 20cc/kg
- Do not insert an intraosseous needle (IO) into a fractured extremity

Secondary Survey

Once the patient is stabilized as above, a thorough examination must be performed as described below. Remember to keep the child warm at all times.

Head

- Basilar skull fracture
    Raccoon eyes = periorbital ecchymosis
    Battle's sign = ecchymosis behind ear
    CSF leak from nose/ears, hemotympanum
- Pupil size, symmetry, and reactivity: unilateral pupil dilatation suggests compression of CN III and possible impending herniation
- Bilateral pupil dilatation is ominous and may suggest severe anoxia/ischemia
- Fundoscopic exam for papilledema as evidence of late increased ICP

Neck

- Cervical spine tenderness, deformities, or injuries
- Trachea midline

Chest

- Clavicle crepitance/tenderness
- Breath sounds
- Heart sounds
- Chest wall movement/symmetry, deformities

Abdomen

- Evaluate for tenderness, distention, bruising
- Shoulder pain may indicate subdiaphragmatic irritation (eg. bleeding)
- Gastric drainage with blood or bile suggests intraabdominal injury
- Left upper quadrant pain, rib tenderness, flank pain may suggest splenic injury

Back

- Asses spine for step-off defects, vertebral tenderness, or open wounds

Extremities

- Check neurovascular status: pulses, perfusion, paresthesias, paralysis, pain
- Check motor/sensory exam
- Check for obvious deformities; focal pain

Neurologic

- A full neurological exam should be performed

NEWBORN RESUSCITATION

Scott J. Cohen, MD[*]

BASIC ALGORITHM

Prior to attending any delivery, all equipment that is necessary and available should be checked and prepared. This includes a warm table, clean and warm towels, oxygen with a bag and mask that is functioning and set appropriately, suction, intubation supplies, catheters, and medications (epinephrine).

Table 1: Factors associated with increased risk for newborn resuscitation

Antepartum Factors	Intrapartum Factors
Maternal age > 35yrs or < 16yrs	Abnormal presentation
Maternal Diabetes	Maternal or fetal infection
Maternal hemorrhage	Prolonged labor
Maternal drug therapy (narcotics; magnesium)	Prolonged rupture of membranes
Maternal substance abuse	Maternal P. Falciparum
Previous fetal/neonatal death	Prolapsed cord
No prenatal care	Meconium-stained fluid
Maternal hypertension	Fetal brady/tachycardia
Maternal anemia	Instrument or C-Section delivery
Fetal malformation noted on ultrasound	Maternal bleeding
Premature rupture of membranes	Precipitous labor
Preterm/post term fetus	Foul-smelling amniotic fluid
Oligohydramnios	
Multiple fetuses	
Maternal illness	
Immature fetal pulmonary studies	

[*] Scott J. Cohen, M.D., Director, Global Pediatric Alliance, Oakland, California

1. Position the baby on a warm surface with a small roll under the scapulae
2. Quickly suction the mouth and nares
3. Dry vigorously the entire body
4. Remove the wet towel
5. Reposition the baby and asses for spontaneous respirations. This is if there is no meconium. If the fluid is meconium-stained, see meconium algorithm below.

If baby is crying at this point, asses color of the lips, and give free-flow oxygen if they appear cyanotic. Asses heart rate and if heart rate is greater than **100/min.**, continue drying and stimulation. For a heart rate less than 100/min., begin positive pressure ventilation. (see below)

RESUSCITATION

If, after doing the initial 5 steps the baby is not crying, then briefly stimulate for 5 seconds by rubbing the spine. If baby still has no spontaneous respirations then resuscitative measures need to be enacted immediately:

Begin positive-pressure ventilation with 100% oxygen for 30 seconds. If oxygen is unavailable, you can use just the bag and mask, or mouth-to-mouth breathing. If mouth-to-mouth breathing is necessary, be sure that the baby's mouth and nose are completely covered by the examiner's mouth. As with all forms of resuscitative ventilation, be sure that the baby's chest rises with each breath. The rate of ventilation should be 1 breath for every 3 seconds.

After the initial 30 seconds of ventilation, if the heart rate is less than 60/min., begin chest compressions (always accompanied by ventilation). Chest compressions should be applied at the intermammary line, on the sternum. The rate of CPR should be 3 compressions followed by 1 ventilation. This should continue for 30 seconds.

After 30 seconds of chest compressions, assess the heart rate. If the heart rate is still less than 60/min., give epinephrine. (see below). If the heart rate is greater than 60/min., stop chest compressions but continue ventilation until there are spontaneous respirations.

EPINEPHERINE

The usual concentration used is 1:1000 solution. Epinephrine can be given via an ETT or intravenously. If Epinephrine is required during a newborn resuscitation, it is best to intubate the baby to secure the airway, and give via the ETT.

Dose

The basic dose is ~0.3cc/kg, which may be repeated every 3-5 minutes as needed. A quick dosing guide is as follows:

- Term infants: 1 cc (of 1:1000)
- Very Large infants: 1.5cc
- Preterm infants: 0.5cc

MECONIUM

When there is meconium-stained amniotic fluid, the following measures are recommended:

- Suction the mouth and nares of the infant when the head is delivered. This should be done before the shoulders are delivered. Suctioning should continue until the secretions are clear. This should be done for both vaginal deliveries and C-sections.
- After the infant is delivered; endotracheal intubation and suctioning should be performed only if the infant does not have spontaneous respirations.
- After tracheal suctioning, the infant should be managed like all other deliveries, beginning with vigorous drying and assessment of breathing.
- Each intubation attempt should be limited to 20 seconds. If intubation is unsuccessful and the infant is bradycardic (heart rate < 100/min.), the infant should receive positive-pressure ventilation until the heart rate is above 100/min. Then another intubation for tracheal suctioning may be attempted.

ENDOTRACHEAL TUBES AND LARYNGOSCOPE

Proper sizing of an endotracheal tube is important to maximize ventilation and avoid damage. The following guidelines may be used to determine size:

- For children less than 8 years of age, an uncuffed tube should be used
- ETT Size = (Age + 16/4)
- Newborns usually use an ETT size of 3.5-4.0
- Depth of insertion (in cm at teeth or lip) is approximately 3 x ETT size
- A straight blade laryngoscope may be used in all ages
- A curved blade may be used in ages 2 and above

APGAR SCORING SYSTEM

Table 2: Apgar Score

Sign	0	1	2
Appearance	Blue throughout	Pink lips/body;blue extremities	Pink lips and body
Pulse Rate	Absent	<100/minute	>100/minute
Grimace	No response to catheter in nares	Some grimace	Cough/sneeze
Activity (Tone)	Limp	Some flexion	Active
Respirations	Absent	Slow irregular	Strong cry

The Apgar scoring system is performed at 1 minute and 5 minutes of life. It is designed to asses with objectivity, the state of health of the immediate newborn infant. Resuscitative measures should not be stopped nor compromised in order to assign the Apgar score.

REFERENCES

1. *John Hopkins: Harriet Lane Handbook*, 15th Ed., 2000, Mosby, St. Louis, pp 420-423
2. Mathers, LH, Frankel, LR, 2000, Stabilization of the Critically Ill Child, *Nelson Textbook of Pediatrics*, W.B. Suanders, Philadelphia, pp 253 - 258

DEHYDRATION IN CHILDREN

Scott J. Cohen, M.D. [*]

DIARRHEA

- Causes 5 - 8 million pediatric deaths/yr.
- Breastfeeding is protective
- Early fluid resuscitation will save lives

SPECIAL CONSIDERATIONS

In early dehydration, the signs and symptoms are subtle, and can lag behind the true state of hydration in the child. As dehydration progresses, clinical signs to look for are: thirst; irritability, decreased activity, drying mucus membranes, absent tears, diminished urine output, increased heart rate. Outcomes are more favorable if fluids can be administered early in the course.

In severe dehydration, these signs are more pronounced, and may include the following: diminished consciousness, anuria, cool extremities, weak pulses or loss of peripheral pulses, sunken fontanel. These are signs of hypovolemic shock, and death may occur if fluids are not started immediately.

ASSESSMENT

History

- Age of patient
- Vomiting? How many times per day? Is the child vomiting just solids, or also clear liquids?
- Diarrhea? How many times per day? Is the diarrhea bloody?

---

[*] Scott J. Cohen, M.D., Director, Global Pediatric Alliance, Oakland, California

- Urine output? (Ideally 1-2cc/kg/hr. The parents should be asked if the child is urinating less than normal, and how many times per day etc.)
- Is the child taking fluids orally? How much?

Physical Exam

The physical exam can be brief and concise. In order to quickly assess degree of dehydration, the exam should focus on the following:

- General state of health and level of consciousness
- Vital signs including heart rate, respiratory rate, temperature, and blood pressure (vital signs are vital). One may also include orthostatic blood pressure in the evaluation of older children
- Absence or presence of tears on exam
- Quality of peripheral pulse
- Capillary refill time
- Warmth or coolness of feet
- Mucus membranes
- Weight loss

Laboratory Studies

If available, basic laboratory studies should be obtained based on the history and physical exam. These may include:

- Complete Blood Count
- Serum Electrolytes, glucose, and BUN/Creatinine
- Bacterial Culture of Stool (if associated with bloody diarrhea or toxic-appearing patient)
- Blood Culture (generally should be reserved for the febrile and toxic-appearing patient)
- Stool for Ova and Parasites (only if suspected)

Table 1: Assessment of Dehydration

Signs and Symptoms	Mild Dehydration	Moderate	Severe
Percent of weight loss	3-5%	6-9%	>10%
Infant Appearance	Thirsty; alert; restless	Thirsty; restless; irritable	Drowsy; limp; cold; sweaty; may be comatose
Child Appearance	Thirsty; alert; restless	Thirsty; alert; orthostatic	Usually conscious; cold; sweaty; tired
Radial Pulse	Normal rate and strength	Rapid and weak	Rapid; impalpable
Respirations		Deep; +/- rapid	Deep and rapid
			Very sunken

Anterior fontanel	Normal	Sunken	Pinch barely retracts
Skin elasticity	Normal turgor	Pinch retracts slowly	Very sunken
Eyes	Normal	Sunken	Absent tears
Tears	Normal	Absent or reduced	Very dry
Mucous membranes	Present	Dry	Severely decreased
Urine output	Slight decrease	Decreased and dark c	> 3 seconds
Capillary refill	Normal	+/- 2 seconds	> 100 cc/kg
Estimated fluid loss	30-50 cc/kg	60-90 cc/kg	

MAINTENANCE FLUID REQUIREMENTS

Table 1: Fluid Requirements

Body Wgt. (kg)	Fluids/ 24 hrs
0 - 10 kg	100cc/kg/24hrs
11 - 20 kg	1000cc + 50cc/kg for each kg body wgt above 10kg
> 20 kg	1500cc + 20cc/kg for each kg body wgt above 20 kg

Examples

- 100cc/kg/day for the 1st 10 kg of body wgt.
- 50cc/kg/day for the 2nd 10 kg of body wgt
- 20cc/kg/day for the 3rd 10 kg of body wgt

TREATMENT

Basic Considerations

- For severe dehydration, circulatory compromise, and/or shock, begin intravenous or intraosseous fluid resuscitation immediately. (see below)
- Parenteral therapy is generally used for severe dehydration, or when a child refuses fluids by mouth, has abdominal distention, or has persistent vomiting.
- For children with mild to moderate dehydration, ORS (oral rehydration solution) may be attempted (either by mouth or nasogastric tube.)
- Children receiving parenteral fluids should be given ORS as soon as they will tolerate orals.

Mild to moderate dehydration

First four hours

- Give 50 - 100cc/kg ORS (Oral Rehydration Solution)
- Try 1 teaspoonful (5cc) for children < 2 yrs every 1-2 minutes;
- Frequent sips from a cup for older children
- If child vomits, wait 10-20 minutes, and resume fluids slowly
- May consider fluids via nasogastric tube if child unable to tolerate orally and no IV available

Remaining 24 hours

- Ideal intake is atleast 100cc/kg/day.
- Children should be encouraged to breastfeed in addition to ORS.
- If child is not vomiting and shows clinical signs of good hydration, can institute feeds with starches and bananas.

Oral Rehydration Solution (ORS)

World Health Organization ORS

- In one litre of clean water
- Glucose 20g
- NaCl 3.5g
- KCl 1.5g
- Trisodium Citrate 2.5g

Homeade ORS

- In 500cc of clean water
- Salt: 3 finger pinch
- Sugar: 4 finger scoop

Alternative Homemade ORS

- In 1 liter of clean water
- 2 Tablespoons of SUGAR or honey
- 1/4 teaspoon SALT
- 1/4 teaspoon BAKING SODA
- Also, add 1/2 cup orange juice, coconut milk, or mashed banana (for potassium)

Severe Dehydration or Shock

Immediate concern should be the restoration of intravascular volume and circulation.

Initial Bolus

Twenty to thirty cc/kg intravenous/intraosseous over 30-45 mins; repeat as often as necessary until hemodynamically stable. (i.e. decreased heart rate, improved cap. refill time, and urine output noted)

- Use Lactated Ringer's or Normal Saline for initial boluses
- Never bolus with dextrose nor potassium in the IV solution
- Most patients with severe dehydration will need 60 - 100cc/ kg to restore volume.
- Monitor urine output and electrolytes
- The severely dehydrated child should be placed on a monitor if available

Maintenance and Deficit

- Easiest way is to give two times maintenance over the first 16 hrs, then 1.5 times maintenance over following 8 hrs.
- IV fluid should contain 1/3 - 1/2 Normal Saline, with 5% Dextrose
- May add KCl (20 mEq/liter) when patient urinates
- May add additional boluses (LR or NS) to replace ongoing losses in diarrhea
- Child should be assessed frequently for signs of improving hydration (see chart on pg. 1)
- Institute ORS when child is ready to tolerate oral fluids
- When signs of dehydration no longer are present, stop IV fluids and begin feeds; continue ORS
- Remember: Once rehydrated and tolerating oral feeds, the best treatment for diarrhea is a bland diet rich in carbohydrates. These may include: breast milk, bananas, steamed rice, plain boiled pasta noodles, baked potatoes, and apple sauce

REFERENCES

1. *Nelson's Textbook of Pediatrics*, 16th Edition; W.B. Saunders Company, Philadelphia, pp 213-215
2. Eddleston M, Pierini S, *Oxford Handbook of Tropical Medicine*. Oxford University Press, 1999

EPIGLOTTITIS

Scott J. Cohen, M.D. & D. James Pyskaty, M.D. [*]

Infectious epiglottitis is one of the most life-threatening pathologic processes involving the airway of a child. Fortunately, its incidence in immunized populations is very low. Epiglottitis occurs in children aged two to seven years, with the peak age being about 3.5 years old. Notably, this is older than the average age for croup. In the U.S., since routine HIB immunization in the late 80's, hemophilus type b is now rarely seen. Non typeable H-flu is seen frequently, but fortunately, this type lacks predilection to infect the epiglottis.

PATHOPHYSIOLOGY

- Predisposition of the organism to infect the epiglottis
- Concurrent bacteremia is common
- Inflammation of the supraglottic tissues rapidly evolves to upper airway edema and poor handling of pharyngeal secretions.

PRESENTATION

- Acute onset of symptoms with very little prodromal illness
- Respiratory distress; begins as little as 6 hours after the initial symptoms
- High fever (often greater than 39)
- Respiratory distress (notably less cough and less stridor than with croup)
- Drooling is present in 60-70 % of patients and is a prominent feature of the illness (because the supraglottic edema precludes effective swallowing of secretions).
- Classic "tripod posture", in which the child prefers to sit forward, resting on both outstretched arms. The neck is hyperextended and the jaw is thrust forward, often with the mouth open and tongue protruding slightly.

[*] Scott J. Cohen, M.D., Director, Global Pediatric Alliance, Oakland, California
D. James Pyskaty, M.D., Assistant Director, Global Pediatric Alliance, Oakland, California

- Anxious and irritable child as the airway edema progresses; this is substantially exacerbated when the child is disturbed in any way.
- Toxic appearance (due to the usual concurrent bacteremia)

Examination of the posterior oropharynx reveals a large, shiny, "cherry-red" epiglottis at the base of the tongue. A lateral neck x-ray will show the pathognomonic "thumb sign", which is the appearance of the epiglottis when substantially inflamed. Normally a thin silhouette, the epiglottis becomes a biconvex structure and the vallecula is obliterated.

TREATMENT

- Rapid stabilization of the airway by an anesthesiologist in the O.R., or the most proficient medical care provider available.
- Intubation is imperative, even if the symptoms seem less than severe.
- While awaiting intubation, the child should be allowed to assume the position of greatest comfort..   The use of racemic epinephrine and corticosteroids are usually ineffective and not routinely recommended.
- Antibiotics (once the airway is stabilized) Ceftriaxone is the most-commonly used, but the combination of ampicillin and chloramphenicol also provides appropriate coverage.
- The usual length of intubation is 2-3 days, during which time, on appropriate antibiotic therapy, the swelling subsides.

Untreated, epiglottitis has a mortality rate of 25%. It is one of the most-urgent airway emergencies for medical practitioners and its diagnosis is often challenging. With appropriate, cautious management, however, the outcome is excellent. Unlike croup, which involves the subglottic structures, epiglottitis is a disease of the supraglottic anatomy.

Table 1: Comparison of Croup and Epiglottitis

	Croup	Epiglottitis
Age	3 months to 3 years	3 – 7 years
Location	Subglottic	Supraglottic
Onset	Gradual	Sudden
Organism	Viral	Bacterial
Fever	100 – 101 F	102 – 104 F
Signs and Symptoms	Barking cough	Drooling
	Retractions	Muffled voice
	Hoarse Voice	Usually no cough
	Harsh cough	Sitting up and leaning
	Loud Stridor	forward; (tripod position)

RESPIRATORY DISEASE IN THE CHILD: EVALUATION AND MANAGEMENT

Scott J. Cohen, MD[*]

EVALUATION

Any respiratory patient showing signs of distress such as tachypnea, tachycardia, retractions, cyanosis, or ill-appearance, will have impending hypoxemia and should be given supplemental oxygen if available. Antibiotics should be considered for an ill-appearing patient who is febrile and/or has focal findings on auscultory exam.

General State of Health

This is perhaps the most important component of evaluating any pediatric patient. The overall appearance of the child is an objective marker of their general state of health. This involves age-appropriate behavior and feeding tolerance. Infants should be able to recognize their parents and be easily consoled, and appear active and vigorous on exam. They should be able to make eye contact with the examiner. Older children should be able to respond appropriately to varying types of interactive stimuli etc.

Respiratory Rate

This is perhaps the single most important piece of data in this evaluation. Tachypnea, a compensatory mechanism, is the most sensitive sign of lower respiratory tract disease in infants and children, and is generally the first sign of respiratory distress. Respirations should be counted for 1 full minute in children under 1 year of age, due to their variable respiratory rate. The examiner should be familiar with normal vital sign values within each age group of children.

---

[*] Scott J. Cohen, M.D., Director, Global Pediatric Alliance, Oakland, California

Heart Rate

Patients with respiratory disease will have tachycardia as a mechanism to increase their cardiac output. This is an early sign of impending hypoxemia. The examiner should measure this vital sign during their evaluations, and be familiar with normal vital sign values in all age groups.

Retractions

Intercostal, subcostal, and supraclavicular retractions are signs of accessory muscle use and represent advancing stages of respiratory distress. Patients should be observed for the presence or absence of these findings.

Auscultation

The patient should be evaluated for degree of aeration, symmetry of breath sounds in all lobes of the lungs, rales, wheezes, and rhonchi.

Mucus membrane

As a late finding in a patient with hypoxemia, the color of the patient's lips and gums may appear cyanotic, or at least less pink than normal.

Oxygen Saturation

Poor oxygen saturations are a late finding in a child with impending hypoxemia. Most children will be ill-appearing, tachycardic, tachypneic, and show retractions before the saturations fall. Therefore, a Pulse-Oxymetry reading should never be used as the sole determinant for administering supplemental oxygen. A good clinical evaluation is the most sensitive guideline.

TRIAGE AND MANAGEMENT

A brief history and physical exam are, of course, an essential part of initial management.

Any apneic patient is dangerously close to cardio-pulmonary collapse and death. They should be resuscitated immediately using an "A.B.C." approach, including endotracheal intubation if indicated.

An unconscious patient, who has spontaneous respirations, should have their airway supported to avoid obstruction. This is best accomplished using the jaw-thrust or chin-lift approach.

Table 1. Principal Causes of Respiratory Distress in Children

Young Infant	Older Infant and Child
Pneumonia	Pneumonia
Bacterial	Bacterial
Viral	Viral
Aspiration	Other
Bronchiolitis	Asthma
Sepsis	Upper Airway Obstruction
Upper Airway Obstruction	Croup
Congenital Heart Disease	Epiglottitis
Intrathoracic Anomalies	Peritonsillar Abscess
Diaphragmatic Hernia	Foreign Body Aspiration
Vascular Rings	Near Drowning
Lobar Empysema	Smoke Inhalation
Cystic Fibrosis	CNS Dysfunction
Infantile Botulism	Pneumothorax
Metabolic Acidosis	Cystic Fibrosis
Dehydration	Neuromuscular disease
Sepsis	Metabolic Acidosis
Inborn errors of metabolism	Diabetic Ketoacidosis
	Toxins

MENINGITIS

Scott J. Cohen, M.D. & D. James Pyskaty, M.D[*].

Meningitis, although rare, is life threatening, and as a result, poses a challenging diagnostic medical problem. The organisms responsible for meningitis depend upon the age of the child, with neonates at risk for infection with *GBS, E. coli* and *Listeria*. After 2 months of age, the organisms most likely to cause meningeal infection change to *H. flu, meningococcus* and *pneumococcus*.

The main epidemiological risks for the disease include young age (with 95% of cases between 1 month and 5 years), splenic dysfunction and proximity to respiratory carriers of the infection. The organisms which cause meningitis are largely transmitted via respiratory droplets. After respiratory droplet inoculation, the infection spreads to the bloodstream, before seeding the meninges. There is evidence that a prior or concurrent viral URI may enhance the pathogenicity of the organism producing the meningitis.

The pathology of meningeal infection includes, often, a meningeal exudative inflammation and a ventriculitis. About 30% of those infected will also have a subdural effusion, often later in the course of the disease. As the cerebral tissue edema progresses and the absorptive arachnoid villae become obstructed, the intracranial pressure of the patient will subsequently rise. Herniation of cerebral structures occurs in 5% of children with infection.

Organisms other than bacteria which can infect the meninges include a wide range of viruses, most commonly the enteroviruses. *Cryptococcus,* syphilis, *HSV, HIV* and cysticercosis represent other less-common causes of aseptic meningitis. One organism which deserves special attention, due to its worldwide prevalence, is tuberculous meningitis – an infection more common in infants and children. The presence of cranial nerve palsies (other than the abducens) with a history of progressive decline in mental status over days to weeks, increases the possibility of tuberculous etiology.

---

[*] Scott J. Cohen, M.D., Director, Global Pediatric Alliance, Oakland, California
D. James Pyskaty, M.D., Assistant Director, Global Pediatric Alliance, Oakland, California

CLINICAL PRESENTATION

- Varies from a subacute, generalized illness to a fulminant toxic illness
- Commonly preceded by several days of an upper respiratory tract infection or gastrointestinal symptoms
- Diagnosis may be complicated by pre-treatment with oral antibiotics (based upon the initial non-specific infectious symptoms resembling a URI or acute otitis media.)
- Non-specific initial symptoms include fever (90-95%), anorexia/ poor feeding, URI and myalgias. (often these are the only symptoms apparent in younger infants)
- Meningeal irritation in older children, (reliably, after 2 years of age):
- These include nuchal rigidity, back pain and photophobia.

Objective signs of meningeal irritation can be screened for by eliciting Kernig's and Brudzinski's signs. Kernig's sign is positive when pain is elicited upon extension of the knee while the hip is in a flexed position. Brudzinski's sign elicits involuntary flexion of the knees and hips following flexion of the neck.

COMPLICATIONS

- SIADH (present in 40% of patients)
- DIC and peripheral gangrene (which is secondary to DIC thrombosis).
- Subdural empyema or cerebral abscess (presents as a relapsing course of illness after appropriate IV antibiotic therapy)
- Neurodevelopmental deficits
- Hearing deficits
- Increased Intracranial Pressure:

Worsening headache, recurrent vomiting, and a bulging fontanel with impending herniation. Cushing's triad includes the concurrent findings of hypertension, bradycardia and apnea. Seizures due to cerebritis are present in 25% of cases of meningitis and are more common with *H. flu* and *pneumococcus*.

DIAGNOSIS

The differential diagnosis for meningitis is somewhat limited because the concerning presence of fever, seizure and toxicity usually prompts immediate assessment for meningeal infection. The benign entity of febrile seizure is, however, one more-common possibility. As a rule, benign febrile seizures are an uncommon occurrence in infants less than 6 months, and therefore, the combination of fever and seizure in this age group should prompt an immediate assessment to rule-out meningitis. Additionally, the diagnosis of benign febrile seizures is similarly rare in children over 5 years old

Definitive diagnosis of meningitis requires a lumbar puncture to identify the etiologic organism. A well equipped microbiology laboratory is essential. As a minimum, gram stain capabilities should be available to analyze the CSF. This invasive procedure is contraindicated when there are signs of increased ICP, severe cardiopulmonary compromise or thrombocytopenia.

If assessment of spinal fluid by LP is delayed yet meningitis is suspected on clinical grounds, empiric antibiotic therapy should be initiated regardless. Presence of >30 leukocytes, or any neutrophil-form predominance implies meningitis, though bacterial infection of the CSF usually produces > 1000 leukocytes. The gram stain is positive in up to 70-90% of patients with disease.

TREATMENT

Antibiotic therapy should be initiated within 30-60 minutes of suspicion of meningitis, due to its potentially rapid course. If the patient is alert, non-lethargic and non-toxic, antibiotics may be safely delayed until CSF studies return. If meningitis is suspected on clinical evaluation, antibiotics should be started empirically even if a lumbar puncture cannot be performed.

- An antibiotic which crosses the blood brain barrier is essential.
- If antibiotic sensitivity profiles are available from the lab, the patient should be switched to the most narrow-spectrum antibiotic when known.
- Ceftriaxone is the most commonly used in the US: (50mg/kg/every 12hrs, or 100mg/kg/every 24 hrs; Adults: 1-2 g/every 12-24 hrs.)
- Cefotaxime is also used widely (50mg/kg/every 6 hrs; Adults: 2g/every 6 hrs)
- A combination of Ampicillin and Chloramphenicol also provide excellent coverage for the most-common organisms. Chloramphenicol may be used alone in penicillin-allergic patients.
      Ampicillin: (50-100mg/kg/every 6 hrs; Adults: 1-3g/every 6 hrs)
      Chloramphenicol: (25mg/kg/every 6 hrs; Adults: 0.5-1g/every 6 hrs)

The use of decadron, given before administration of antibiotics, should be considered, if the organism is *H.flu*. There is some evidence that this combination may decrease inflammation and hearing deficits.

Post-treatment prophylaxis of the patient and intimate contacts is critical to eradicate nasal carriage of *H. flu* and *meningococcus*. Rifampin or Ciprofloxacin, if available, is recommended.

The maintenance of cerebral perfusion is critical ancillary management for the process. This perfusion pressure maintains adequate blood flow to the brain.
Excessive intracranial pressure can contribute to a risk for ongoing obtundation and potential herniation of brain matter. Additional therapy for complications of meningeal inflammation includes fluid restriction for signs of SIADH and treatment of seizures with ativan and potentially dilantin.

DURATION OF THERAPY

- *H.influenza type B*   7 -10 days
- *Streptococcal pneumoniae*   10 -14 days
- *N. meningitidis*   7 days
- *E. coli*   21 days
- *Group B Strep.*   14 - 21 days
- *Listeria*   14 - 21 days

PROGNOSIS

The prognosis for a patient with meningitis is variable and depends greatly upon the rapidity of diagnosis and initiation of treatment. Even with timely therapy, severe neurodevelopmental sequelae arise in 15% of patients and mild neurobehavioral irregularities are ultimately seen in over half. These sobering facts accent the need for prompt, thoughtful diagnosis and appropriate therapy without delay.

REFERENCES

1. Prober CG, Central Nervous System Infections, *Nelson Textbook of Pediatrics*, *16th Ed.*, W.B. Saunders, Philadelphia, pp 751-757

PLASMODIUM FALCIPARUM MALARIA IN CHILDREN

Scott J. Cohen, M.D.[*]

Plasmodium falciparum malaria remains a major global health threat to children. Along with respiratory disease, dehydration, measles and malnutrition, malaria is one of the top five killers of children in the tropics. The increasing occurrence of drug resistance only exacerbates this tragedy.

Severe malaria in children, especially under 5 years of age, can develop quite rapidly and progress to multi-system organ disease if prompt diagnosis and treatment are not instituted. Any child, who is febrile in an area endemic for malaria, should be tested for this infection. If no diagnostic facilities are available, then empiric therapy should be instituted. If facilities are available for thick and thin smears then a febrile child who is ill appearing, should be started on anti-malarial treatment while awaiting laboratory results.

The diagnosis of malaria in children may be difficult. Many of the symptoms may represent other diseases. Also, many children have a baseline parasitemia, which may be clinically insignificant relative to their presenting symptoms. Fever may be variable and not synchronized; vomiting and diarrhea may represent an intestinal infection. Many causes of anemia are present in the tropics and may not necessarily be from malaria. And, febrile seizures, hypoglycemia, epilepsy, and bacterial meningitis may all mimic the presentation of cerebral malaria.

Although any child may be vulnerable to all of the complications of severe malaria seen in adults, the 4 most common complications in children will be discussed in this chapter. They are as follows: cerebral malaria, severe anemia, metabolic acidosis (presenting as respiratory distress), and hypoglycemia

MANAGEMENT

[*] Scott J. Cohen, M.D., Director, Global Pediatric Alliance, Oakland, California

General principles

- Assess Airway, Breathing, Circulation (always)
- Vital Signs
- Assess level of consciousness and general state of health
- Assess level of hydration
- Check blood sugar immediately
- Thick and thin films
- Hemoglobin or hematocrit
- Consider lumbar puncture for bacterial meningitis

Immediate Interventions

- Airway, Breathing, and Circulation resuscitation if warranted
- Treat seizures
- Correct hypoglycemia
- Restore intravascular volume
- Nasogastric tube if child is unconscious
- Begin empiric treatment for P. Falciparum
- Treat fever
- Consider empiric antibiotic treatment

Table 1: Differences between adults and children with Plasmodium falciparum

Sign or Symptom	Adults	Children
History of Cough	Uncommon	Common
Seizures	Common	Very common
Duration of illness	5 -7 days	1-2 days
Resolution of coma	2 -4 days	1-2 days
Neurological sequelae	<5%	>10%
Jaundice	Common	Uncommon
Pulmonary edema	Uncommon	Rare
Renal failure	Common	Uncommon
Pretreatment hypoglycemia	Uncommon	Common
CSF opening pressure	Usually normal	Usually raised
Respiratory distress	Sometimes	Common
Abnormal brain stem reflexes	Rare	Somewhat common
Bleeding problems	Up to 10%	Rare

CEREBRAL MALARIA

Clinical Presentation

- Fever, decreased activity, refusing food or drink, emesis
- Brief period of 1-2 days prodromal symptoms prior to <u>coma</u>
- Seizures, nystagmus, salivation, myoclonic activity
- Hypoperfusion, cold extremities, shock

Management

- See "Immediate Interventions" above
- Meticulous nursing care
    - Nurse patient in lateral position to avoid aspiration
    - Manage nasogastric tube
    - Turn patient every 2 hours to prevent bed sores
    - Strict records intake and output
    - Monitor urine volume, specific gravity, and asses for hemoglobinuria
    - Meticulous attention to IV fluid rate to avoid overly rapid infusions
    - Vital signs and Glasgow coma scale assessment every 4 hours
    - Fever reduction with fans, tepid sponging, and medications
- Monitor blood glucose every 4-8 hours
- Packed red blood cell transfusion if severe anemia present

SEVERE ANEMIA

Clinical Presentation

- Assess effect of anemia on clinical presentation, rather than an absolute hemoglobin value
- A rapid drop in RBC's from a high parasitemia will result in:
    - Shock/ Circulatory collapse
    - Metabolic Acidosis and respiratory distress from hypoxemia

Management

- Generally, a child who presents with a hemoglobin level of < 4.5gm/dl should be transfused with 10-15cc/kg of packed red blood cells immediately
- A child with a hemoglobin level of 4-6 gm/dl and shows signs of circulatory compromise, respiratory distress, impaired consciousness, or high parasitemia (>20%), should be transfused immediately

METABOLIC ACIDOSIS/ RESPIRATORY DISTRESS

Clinical Presentation

- Tachypnea

- Intercostal and subcostal retractions
- Circulatory compromise/ shock

Management

- Secure intravenous or intraosseous line
- Correct cause of acidosis:
    Dehydration
    Anemia
    Shock
- Bolus 20cc/kg of Saline as needed to restore circulating volume
- Packed red blood cell transfusion as indicated
- Close and serial monitoring of level of consciousness, hydration, anemia, and blood glucose

HYPOGLYCEMIA

Clinical Presentation

- Common in children under age 3 yrs. with malaria
- Commonly associated with seizures, hyperparasitemia, and coma
- Easily overlooked as may mimic symptoms of cerebral malaria

Management

- 0.5gm/kg IV of Dextrose: (5cc/kg of D10W) (Dextrose 10g/100cc soln.)
- Give initial bolus over ~10-15 minutes
- Maintenance infusion of 5% dextrose should follow initial bolus, to prevent further hypoglycemia
- May give via nasogastric tube if parenteral routes unavailable
- Serial monitoring of blood glucose levels

PHARMACOLOGIC TREATMENT OF *P. FALCIPARUM* MALARIA

If IV Treatment Possible

- Loading Dose: 20mg/kg Quinine IV diluted in 10mg/kg Normal Saline or 5% Dextrose; give over 4-6hrs.
- Do not give loading dose if child received quinine, quinidine, or mefloquine in past 12hrs
- Maintenance Dose: 12 hours after loading dose infused, give Quinine 10mg/kg IV, infused over 2 hrs. Repeat this dosing every 12 hours.
- When patient can tolerate PO's, give Quinine 10mg/kg (600mg max.) every 8 hrs to complete a 7day course.

If IV Treatment Not Possible

- Loading Dose: 20mg/kg quinine diluted in 60mg/ml Saline; inject IM in thighs
- Maintenance Dose: 10mg/kg IM every 12 hrs until able to take oral meds

If No Parenteral Treatment Possible

- Quinine tablets 10mg/kg by mouth or nasogastric tube every 8 hours to complete 7-day course
- Refer to higher level of care if possible

Alternative Oral Regimens

- Sulfadoxine 25mg/kg, and pyrimethamine 1.25mg/kg, single oral dose after 3 days of quinine
- Mefloquine 15mg/kg orally, single dose; then 10mg/kg orally in 24 hrs if patient remains ill

REFERENCES

1. Management of Severe Malaria; A Practical Handbook
   World Health Organization, 2nd Edition, 2000
2. O'Dempsey, Tim. *Malaria in Children*. Africa Health (supplement). Sept. 2000;
   21-26
3. Bell, Dion; Tropical Medicine. Blackwell Science, Ltd. 4th Edition. 1995

ETHICAL ISSUES IN PEDIATRIC RESUSCITATION

Deirdre M. Fearon, Ed.M, M.D.*

An estimated 25,745 children died in the United States in 2000. The leading causes of death were unintentional injury, Sudden Infant Death Syndrome, drowning, poisoning, choking, asthma, and pneumonia. Many of these children present to the emergency department (ED) in cardiopulmonary arrest. The American Heart Association recommends attempting resuscitation unless there is a valid Do Not Attempt Resuscitation order or signs of irreversible death, such as dependent lividity, decapitation, or rigor mortis. It is difficult to predict which individual patients will have favorable outcomes, but there are several prognostic factors predictive of survival to hospital discharge. These include: a palpable pulse on presentation, a short interval between arrest and hospital arrival, fewer doses of epinephrine, and short duration of resuscitation in the ED. Without return of spontaneous circulation after 30 minutes of ACLS, the chance of survival is exceedingly small.

Emergency physicians face unique challenges compared to other physicians. Decisions must be made quickly and with incomplete data, emotions in the resuscitation room frequently run high, and the prognosis of acutely ill patients is often unclear. In addition, parents are frequently absent upon a child's initial presentation. Even when parents are available, they have no established relationship with the emergency physician. Difficult, important decisions must, therefore, be made without prior knowledge of the family's values.

These practical challenges add to the complexity of the many ethical questions that arise in the setting of pediatric resuscitation. Several of these present a particular ethical challenge to the emergency physician, including:

1. When are resuscitation attempts futile, and is the ED physician obligated to provide futile care at the family's insistence?

---

* Deirdre M. Fearon, Ed.M, M.D., Department of Pediatrics and Section of Emergency Medicine
Brown Medical School, Pediatric Emergency Medicine, Hasbro Children's Hospital
Providence, Rhode Island

2. What if the family has religious objections to either providing or withholding care?
3. Should the family be present in the resuscitation room?
4. Can procedures be practiced on the recently deceased child without permission from the parents?
5. Can resuscitation research be performed without informed consent?

In the bioethics literature, these and other questions are often addressed with the principles of autonomy, beneficence, nonmalificence, and justice in mind. Autonomy refers to a person's ability to make his or her own decisions or decisions for his/her children; beneficence is doing good; nonmalificence is the principle that describes the credo, "first, do no harm"; and justice is the notion that everyone be treated fairly. There are times in the practice of medicine when these principles are competing. For example, respecting a patient's decision to refuse care may cause that patient physical harm. These circumstances -- when there appear to be equally compelling ethical arguments for mutually exclusive courses of action -- are ethical dilemmas. Some of the ethical dilemmas faced in the pediatric resuscitation room will be addressed in this chapter.

FUTILITY

Both ethicists and physicians have offered many different definitions of futility, but they all share the general notion that an act is futile when there is virtually no chance of achieving the desired goal using the means available. Within this definition, there are both quantitative and qualitative components. Quantitative questions in pediatric resuscitation include: what is the probability of survival out of the ED, of survival out of the hospital, and of life without neurological sequelae. The qualitative questions, which by definition are value-laden, are those surrounding the goals of the involved parties.

There is no consensus about the goals of medicine, but they generally concern the relief of suffering, prolongation of life, and the maintenance or restoration of good health. Additionally, physicians maintain the goal of allocating resources fairly to patients. Physicians also have the wish to maintain professional integrity, i.e. they want to act in ways that avoid injury to their own self-images both as a people and as professionals. Parents have goals as well, both for their children and for themselves. They generally want to avoid painful procedures for their children and to provide them with a good quality of life. Parents also want to have their children live as long as possible, and they want to maintain their autonomy as decision-makers for their children.

The dilemma in the case of futility is what to do when parents insist that the physician "do everything" when the physician feels that nothing he/she does will be of any benefit or may even be injurious to the patient. Physicians want to respect parents as autonomous decision-makers for their children but also want to practice good medicine. Do physicians have the right to refuse to provide care they believe is futile?

Those in favor of physicians being obligated to "do everything" in this circumstance emphasize the parents' right to make decisions for their child. Parents have a unique knowledge as to the needs of their children as well as their own ability to care for their children. Parents have made every other decision about how to raise the child and have his or her best interest in mind. Why should they not be allowed to make this final decision about their child's care? Additionally, some might argue that this particular child could be the one in a million to defy "futility" and do well. There is, after all, some degree of prognostic uncertainty in resuscitation.

While these are convincing arguments in favor of parents having a strong voice in decision-making, there are several persuasive arguments in favor of the physician not being obliged to provide care he/she sees as futile. Physicians have medical expertise after years of training and with knowledge of current data, should have a good idea of who will survive resuscitation with a positive outcome. They are the medical experts and should know what the best course of action is in a given setting.

Another argument against of provision of futile care is that of distributive justice. Each patient in the ED has a right to excellent care. If the ED physician spends hours attempting to resuscitate an infant who will surely not survive, other sick children may receive sub-optimal care.

Some physicians may cite resident education or staff practice as a reason for proceeding with a futile resuscitation. This is essentially performing procedures on the recently deceased, a topic that will be addressed later in the chapter. Others indicate that they go through the motions for the family. They want to be able to tell the family that everything possible was done for their child. The physician wants to do what is best for the family, and they are willing to sacrifice some of the parents' autonomy to do so. This situation -- when beneficence overrides autonomy -- is paternalism. This is justified only if the family is incapable of acting in their own best interest at the moment. There is no reason to believe that, as a rule, parents of very sick children are unable to act in their own best interest. Paternalism and deceit are not justified in this situation. Parents are generally competent decision makers and should be respected enough to be told the truth.

A final, poignant argument in support of physicians withholding futile care is that physicians are also moral agents, not merely technicians who make themselves available to carry out parental wishes. Surely, no one would expect a neurosurgeon to perform a lobotomy simply because a mother requested one for her child. Similarly, the ED physician is not obligated to perform care that does not meet with the professional standards of emergency medicine. If a child is not revived after 30 minutes of ACLS or multiple doses of epinephrine, the ED physician -- knowing the dismal prognosis -- should not be obligated to continue, even if parents insist.

The American Academy of Emergency Physicians released a policy statement in 1998 stating, "Physicians are under no ethical obligation to render treatments that they judge to have no realistic likelihood of benefiting the patient." This seems true given the previous arguments. However, the ED physician should always attempt to include families in decision-making and should continue to acknowledge medical uncertainty, erring on the side of attempting to revive the child.

PARENTS IN THE RESUSCITATION ROOM

The classic scene of a parent being physically escorted from a resuscitation room by a nurse has been called into question in recent years, although this longstanding practice still occurs in many hospitals. Physicians and nurses often feel anxious with parents in the room and worry that their presence may serve as a distraction from the resuscitation itself. Others worry that parents may interfere with the resuscitation or demand that efforts continue past a reasonable point. Even if parents quietly observe, medical staff worry about the psychological effect of witnessing what can be a somewhat harsh series of events.

While the intentions of ED staff may be well intentioned, protecting parents from their own decisions is paternalistic and disrespectful of parental autonomy. There is enough trauma room television for people to have some appreciation of what to expect. Doctors and nurses can also prepare parents about tube placement and line insertions. Parents must be respected as competent decision-makers about their own desire and ability to observe the resuscitation attempt. Occasionally, a hysterical parent may attempt to interfere, but this relatively rare occurrence can quickly be handled if it presents itself.

Surveys have shown that most parents wish to be with their child during procedures, even in major resuscitations that will likely end with the death of the child. Parents have also reported an easier bereavement process after they saw what was done in an effort to save their child. If children do survive, having a parent in the room may serve as a comfort.

Doctors must be honest about why they do not want parents in the room. If it is so that the least qualified person can attempt procedures or so that people do not have to converse in a professional manner, they should consider the fact that these practices are inappropriate, regardless of who observes them. If an intern performs the intubation, it should be with direct supervision whether parents are present or not. And though tension and pressure may lead to less sensitive dialogue, even unconscious patients should always be shown respect.

The evidence indicates that having parental presence in the trauma room is good for parents and generally not detrimental to the procedure. Parents may be hesitant to ask to be present and should, therefore, be explicitly offered that opportunity. As a rule, a support person should be assigned to the parent to explain procedures and answer questions.

PROCEDURES ON THE NEWLY DEAD

In about half of ED's that serve as training sites for residents, the newly dead are used to teach and practice procedures. Endotracheal intubation is most commonly performed as well as central line placement, cricothyrotomy, thoracotomy, cut-downs and chest tube placement. Considerable discussions have occurred around whether or not consent should be obtained prior to using these cadavers for teaching. Generally, consent is not obtained from the patient or his/her surviving family members prior to practicing procedures on the deceased. There are valid arguments for both requiring consent and performing the procedures without consent.

Those who argue against the necessity of obtaining consent insist that dead people cannot be harmed, that society expects and benefits from proficiency and that animal and mannequin models are inadequate substitutes for learning procedures to be performed on humans. The alternative is to learn these skills on the living, in the operating room, often without their knowledge or explicit consent, or on a living person in the midst of resuscitation. Practically speaking, obtaining consent from surviving family members to do procedures on a recently deceased person is awkward and often the family is not immediately available. Proponents of a no-consent policy appeal to "presumed consent" – the notion that consent can be assumed if a reasonable person would consent to the procedure in similar circumstances.

Those in favor of requiring consent appeal to autonomy arguments, stating that the deceased did not consent to any of these procedures and thus, they should not be performed. A counter argument to this is that the deceased are no longer persons and, therefore, have no autonomy. However, this argument seems weak when we consider how the dead are treated in our culture. Dead bodies must be respected, i.e. shouldn't be mutilated or left in the street. And even when someone is dead, his or her will must be respected. The deceased is no longer able to express a wish, but those wishes expressed before death should be respected.

The next of kin have the right to make decisions regarding the body of the deceased through quasi-property rights.   Thus, they have a responsibility to make decisions regarding cremation or burial.   And with that responsibility comes the right to make decisions about non-therapeutic procedures performed on the body. The family members have a valid claim to the body; the medical staff has none.

It is important to recall that any sort of medical touching without consent is considered battery. While implied consent is assumed in an emergency, that consent is for care that will benefit the patient.   The unconscious, vulnerable patient is not necessarily consenting for procedures to be performed that are not done in an effort to help him or her. Similarly, parental permission is assumed for a child in an emergency situation but only for potentially beneficial care, not for experimentation.

Some might argue that each person has an obligation to future resuscitation patients to allow practice procedures to be performed post-mortem. While it would be a kind and generous act, our society does not require altruism. In our culture, we respect each other's right to be left alone and cannot make moral demands on others, particularly when those demands infringe on the rights and desires of those same people upon whom the demands are made.

Available data suggest that most patients would allow procedures to be practiced on their loved ones if asked. It is a difficult question for physicians to ask at a very difficult time. But if phrased correctly, the survivors may find some comfort in helping others, even in their own time of loss. As physicians, it is important to consider how we would want our loved ones treated and if we want to be included in those decisions.

RELIGIOUS OJECTIONS TO CARE

Jehovah's Witnesses and Christian Scientists are two of the most widely known religious groups who refuse at least some medical care. Jehovah's Witnesses interpret the Bible literally, including verses that prohibit blood consumption. They interpret this as not just a prohibition of oral consumption but taking blood into the body in any way. For Witnesses, to break this rule is to give up a chance at eternal life. Christian Scientists believe that healing is done through prayer. They will often pray over a sick child before seeking medical consultation and may not present to an ED until the child is very sick. Even then, the Christian Science parent may wish for as little medical intervention to be done as possible.

In these cases, there are several conflicting rights. Parents generally have the right to make medical decisions for their children. Children have a right to life and adequate health care, and physicians have the right to practice in accordance with medical standards of care. The law is clear here; parents cannot put their children at risk of death or serious harm for religious reasons. A 1944 court ruling unrelated to medical care stated, "Parents may be free to become martyrs themselves, but it does not follow that they are free to make martyrs of their children."

The ethical obligation of the physician is clear as well: he/she must do what is in the best interest of the patient. Generally, doing what is in the best interest of the family is also good for the child because of the intimate relationship between children and parents. There are times though when respecting the family's wishes puts the child in danger of serious harm or death. In these circumstances, the family's wishes must be overruled by what is best for the child.

If compromises can be found and the child is not put at serious risk, alternatives should be attempted first. For example, if a child of a Jehovah's Witness presents with blood loss, initial attempts at volume expansion with saline can be attempted first if the patient is stable. If the parents' wishes cannot ultimately be honored and time permits, a court order should be obtained. However, if the child is in grave danger, appropriate care should be provided while a court order is being requested.

RESUSCITATION RESEARCH

From a pathophysiologic perspective, relatively little is known about the science of pediatric resuscitation. Thankfully, pediatric cardiac arrest is a rare event; however, that relative infrequency makes performing large studies of pediatric resuscitation so difficult.

Generally, informed consent for research is impractical to obtain in the resuscitation room. Often parents are unavailable or when they are present, the resuscitation itself must take precedent over time spent carefully explaining research aims and obtaining signatures. The Department of Health and Human Services, in conjunction with the

National Institutes of Health, addressed this important issue in 1996 by allowing a waiver of the need to obtain informed consent in limited circumstances.

When designing resuscitation research studies, strict guidelines must be followed. The potential benefit to the patient, the expected safety of the protocol, and the possible benefit to society must all be considered. Both expert and community consultation must be sought, including a review of the study by a local Institutional Review Board. In addition, there must be public disclosure of the nature of the research within the effected community.

RECOMMENDATIONS

1. Keep current with resuscitation research in order to make the most informed decisions possible.
2. Strongly consider stopping resuscitation if there is no return of spontaneous circulation after 30 minutes of ACLS.
3. Keep parents involved. Invite them into the resuscitation room with a support person. Try to involve them in important decisions. Be respectful of their opinions, but keep the well being of the child top priority.
4. Physicians are not obliged to provide inappropriate or futile care. Recognize that parents and physicians may place different value on survival with severe neurological sequelae, and may, therefore, define futility differently.
5. Respect the deceased and the families of the deceased. Attempt to obtain consent before performing procedures on the newly dead.

Pediatric resuscitation is one of the most difficult aspects of emergency medicine. Everyone wants desperately to keep children alive and help parents avoid tremendous loss. Considering these difficult ethical questions ahead of time may allow the emergency physician to stay more focused in the flurry of a resuscitation situation. Well thought out beliefs can keep the physician from making decisions he/she may later regret, and enable him/her to run a resuscitation optimally for both the child and the family.

REFERENCES

1. Abramson N, de Vos R, Fallat ME, et al. Ethics in emergency cardiac care. Annals of Emergency Medicine 2001; 37:S196-200.
2. ACEP Policy Statement. Ethical Issues for Resuscitation. Dallas, TX, 2001.
3. ACEP Policy Statement. Nonbeneficial ("futile") emergency medical interventions. American College of Emergency Physicians Dallas, TX, 1998.
4. Adams S, Whitlock M, Higgs R, Bloomfield P, Baskett PJF. Should relatives be allowed to watch resuscitation? British Medical Journal. 1994; 308: 1687-1689.
5. American Academy of Pediatrics Committee on Bioethics. Religious objections to medical care. Pediatrics 1997; 99:279-81.
6. American Academy of Pediatrics Committee on Bioethics. Ethics and the Care of Critically Ill Infants and Children (RE9624). Pediatrics 1996; 98(1): 149-152.
7. Boie ET, Moore GP, Brummett C, Nelson DR. Do parents want to be present during invasive procedures performed on their children in the emergency department? A survey of 400 parents. Pediatrics 1997; 99:279-81.

8. Boyd R. Witnessed resuscitation by relatives. Resuscitation. 2000; 43: 171-176.
9. Department of Health and Human Services, Food and Drug Administration: Protection of human subjects; informed consent and waiver of informed consent requirements in certain emergency research final rules. Federal Register FR Doc. 96-24968, 9/26/96.
10. Davies JM, Reynolds BM. The ethics of cardiopulmonary resuscitation. I. Background to decision making. Archives of Disease in Childhood. 1992; 67: 1498-1501.
11. Davies JM, Reynolds BM. The ethics of cardiopulmonary resuscitation. II. Medical logistics and the potential for good response. Archives of Disease in Childhood. 1992; 67: 1502-1505.
12. Doyle CJ, Post H, Burney RE, Maino J, Keefe M, Rhee KJ. Family participation during resuscitation: an option. Annals of Emergency Medicine. 1987; 16: 673-675.
13. Fontanarosa PB, Giorgio GT. The role of the emergency physician in the management of Jehovah's Witnesses. Annals of Emergency Medicine 1989; 18:1089-95.
14. Fourre MW. The Performance of Procedures on the Recently Deceased. Academic Emergency Medicine 2002; 9:595-598.
15. Forman EN, Ladd RE. Ethical Dilemmas in Pediatrics. A Case Study Approach. University Press of America Inc. 1995. Lanham, MD.
16. Goldblatt AD. Don't ask, don't tell: practicing minimally invasive resuscitation techniques on the newly dead. Annals of Emergency Medicine 1995; 25:91-4.
17. Hanson C, Strawser D. Family presence during cardiopulmonary resuscitation: Foote Hospital emergency department's nine-year perspctive. Journal of Emergency Nursing. 1992; 18: 104-106
18. Hoyert DL, Freedman MA, Strobino DM, Guyer B. Annual summary of vital statistics: 2000. Pediatrics 2001; 108:1241-55.
19. Iserson KV. Law versus life: the ethical imperative to practice and teach using the newly dead emergency department patient. Annals of Emergency Medicine 1995; 25:91-94.
20. Jonsen AR. Blood transfusions and Jehovah's Witnesses. The impact of the patient's unusual beliefs in critical care. Critical Care Clinics 1986; 2:91-100.
21. Luce JM. Physicians do not have a responsibility to provide futile or unreasonable care if a patient or family insists. Critical Care Medicine 1995; 23(4): 760-766.
22. Manifold CA, Storrow A, Rodgers K. Patient and family attitudes regarding the practice of procedures on the newly deceased. Acad Emerg Med. 1999; 6:110-115.
23. Marco CA. Determination of "futility" in emergency medicine. [letter; comment.] [erratum appears in Acad Emerg Med 2000 Aug;36(2):171.]. Annals of Emergency Medicine 2000; 35.
24. Marco CA. Ethical issues of resuscitation. Emergency Medicine Clinics of North America 1999; 17:527-38.
25. Marco CA. Research ethics: ethical issues of data reporting and the quest for authenticity. [see comments.]. Emergency Medicine Clinics of North America 1999; 17:527-38.
26. May L. Challenging medical authority. The refusal of treatment by Christian Scientists. [see comments.]. Hastings Center Report 1995; January-February:15-21.
27. Nichols DG, Kettrick RG, Swedlow DB, Lee S, Passman R, Ludwig S. Factors influencing outcome of cardiopulmonary resuscitation in children. Pediatric Emergency Care 1986; 2: 1-5.
28. Patterson MD. Resuscitation update for the pediatrician. Pediatric Clinics of North America 1999; 46:1285-303.
29. Prince v. Com. of Mass., 321 U.S. 158 (1944)
30. Robinson SM, Mackenzie-Ross S, Campbell Hewson GL, Egleston CV, Prevost AT. Psychological effect of witnessed resuscitation on bereaved relatives. Lancet 1998; 352: 614-617.
31. Schindler MB, Bohn D, Cox PN, et al. Outcome of out-of-hospital cardiac or respiratory arrest in children. The New England Journal of Medicine 1996; 335:1473-1479.
32. The American Heart Association in collaboration with the International Liaison Committee on Resuscitation. Guidelines 2000 for Cardiopulmonary Resuscitation and Emergency Cardiovascular Care. Part 2: Ethical Aspects of CPR and ECC. Circulation 2000; 102:II2-21.
33. Truog RD, Brett AS, Frader J. The Problem With Futility. New England Journal of Medicine 1992; 326:1560-1563.
34. Tsai E. Should family members be present during cardiopulmonary resuscitation? New England Journal of Medicine 2002; 346:1019-21.

HIGH RISK ACUTE CARE

Lawrence Proano, M.D.[*]

In the 1990s emergency physicians have come under increasing scrutiny in the performance of their profession. This problem is ongoing in the United States and may soon be the subject of intense government scrutiny, monitoring and regulation. In the past decade jury awards for malpractice suits have continued to increase, with seemingly no ceiling in sight.

There is a heightened awareness by the public of the concept of medical error and a specific focus by emergency physicians to reduce errors in emergency care. Emergency medicine is recognized as a specialty with one of the greatest exposures for physicians to situations involving life threatening conditions requiring critical decision making.

This chapter is a review of some of the most high risk aspects of care in emergency medicine. It is focused on improving quality of care and raising the awareness of concepts of risk management for clinicians. This is presented with a goal to decrease medical errors and improve outcomes or patients presenting to emergency care facilities.

FACTORS PROMOTING LITIGATION

Several factors come into play which promotes the filing of malpractice claims. One of these is the heightened expectations patients have of the care they receive and the outcome they will experience in the course of treatment of their condition.

Rapid progression of technology has fostered some of this expectation. With advancements in medical care the bar has been raised in the standard of care for treatment of emergency conditions. Technology has brought more rapid dissemination of information to society. This wave of "consumerism" has spilled over to the delivery of medical care as well.

---

[*] Lawrence Proano, M.D., Associate Professor, Brown University/Rhode Island Hospital, Department of Emergency Medicine, Providence, Rhode Island

Emergency medicine practice often has its own specific shortfalls that increase the potential to produce an unhappy patient even in the most straightforward circumstances. The emergency department is generally a strange environment for the patient and their family members. Typically, the waiting areas are small and uncomfortable areas, and the waits can be very prolonged.

This all likely occurs in a setting of a stressful situation, depending on the extent of the patient's illness or injury. In addition, the patient by being sent to a treatment area, and their loved ones, sent to the waiting room, are often thus separated during the specific time when they would normally be together in a supportive fashion in most other stressful life situations. These environmental and logistical factors all work to increase, rather than decrease, anxiety in patients and their families.

Yet another factor that works to the disadvantage of the clinician in the fact that the patient likely does not know them, as they might know their primary care family physician. This effect of not having a prior bond or relationship with the emergency physician makes the patient much more likely to want to place blame in the event of an untoward event. This may be true even if there is no causal link to the physician's treatment and the outcome incurred.

Even in the face of perfect medical care, all these factors work against the emergency physician's efforts to reduce their risk of exposure to malpractice claims. Therefore, emergency physicians must change their practice to counter these factors in their approach to patients and their families.

The final common denominator comes down to setting the stage for the medical encounter and through proper communication. The physician should work to create and nurture the best relationship possible during the brief period they have with their patient. Social science studies have demonstrated that the impression a person has of a physician is distinctly influenced by the physician's behavior and demeanor during that encounter.

For example, studies have revealed that a common recurring complaint is that patients don't feel their physician has spent sufficient time with them. A simple maneuver such as sitting during the interview has been demonstrated to cause patients of feel that more time was spent with them, versus the same amount of time spent in a standing position.

Similarly, studies have suggested that how the family feels about the experience in emergency care of a patient is as much an influence in the filing of a malpractice claim as is the impression of the patient themselves. Family members have a great deal of influence in patient decisions to file lawsuits. The experience of the family with the physician and the institution is thus a very important factor in this regard.

Despite these psychosocial factors, the most common reason for malpractice suits in medicine is still that of genuinely negligent acts of commission or omission. Many of these are avoidable. In November 1999, the Institute of Medicine (IOM) issued a report on medical error, To Err is Human: Building a Safer Health System. Their study suggested that as many as 100,000 patients die annually in the U.S. from medical error.

The exact figure is controversial, but the general concept remains that error in medicine is a problematic issue, and this includes the specialty of emergency medicine.

SURVEYING THE MEDICOLEGAL LANDSCAPE

In order for emergency physicians to be able to make inroads into the litigation crisis, it is important for them to examine the myriad entities which one encounters in an active practice of emergency medicine. In the United States there have been efforts to try to identify those areas of highest risk malpractice.

Several closed claims studies have been done in this regard. In the mid 1980's, the American College of Emergency physicians sponsored and conducted such a study. It illustrated that a limited number of entities could be identified which would account for the vast majority of malpractice claims filed (Table 1).

Table 1: Close Claim Data

Failure to Diagnose	Percent of Cases	Percent of Dollars Paid
Fracture	27.4	13.5
Foreign body in a wound	13.8	4.2
Tendon/nerve complications	13.6	5.6
Myocardial infarction	10.2	31.8
Appendicitis	4.8	4.5
Meningitis	2.3	15.4
Skull/facial fracture	2.3	2.9
Ectopic pregnancy	2.0	8.2
Intraabdominal Injuries	1.2	2.0
All others	21.6	11.9

Similarly the Massachusetts Medical Society performed a detailed closed claims study over a three year period form 1988-1990. They reviewed 262 claims processed by the state mandated carrier. This study revealed that $11,800,156 in claims were paid out in awards and settlements during this period.

There were 211 cases that represented a failure to diagnose a specific entity. Of these 211 cases, 184 fell into only 8 categories. These included chest pain, abdominal pain, wounds, fractures, aortic aneurysms, epiglottitis, central nervous system (CNS) bleeds, and the febrile child. The awards and settlements from these eight groups constituted 66% of the total payout for all the 262 claims during the study period.

BASIC MEDICOLEGAL CONCEPTS

A basic working knowledge of legal medicine is also helpful to the emergency physician in being able to understand some of the basic concepts and the process by which malpractice actions take place. One of these concepts is understanding the four elements required in order to file a lawsuit for negligence:

- A duty to treat
- A breach in the standard of care
- An injury to the patient
- A causal link demonstrated between the breach and the injury

The term "standard of care" for emergency medicine is particularly important to understand if it is to be met. It can be defined as the degree of care that a reasonably prudent emergency physician would exercise under the same or similar circumstance. If it can be demonstrated that an emergency physician did not provide the kind of care which most reasonably prudent emergency physicians would give in a specific scenario for a specific entity, then one of the elements necessary to file a claim has been met.

In general, the reasons physicians fail to meet the standard of care in medicine, and in emergency medicine specifically, fall into two primary categories- a deficit in their knowledge base, or despite an adequate knowledge base a gap in clinical performance.

Thus, the cornerstone of any personal or departmental plan or program in risk management or risk reduction must remain the delivery of high quality medical care. By incorporating these concepts into ones practice, it is far easier to protect oneself in the face of an unfriendly medico legal climate.

GENERAL PITFALLS

Some recurrent general error themes can be identified in clinical practice which contribute to the generation of untoward results and in malpractice claims. Among these are:
- Failure to note or address abnormal vital signs
- Inadequate exam in the intoxicated patient
- Failure to address nursing notes (or ambulance reports)
- Failure to document wellness on the medical record
- Failure to get high risk patients seen quickly
- Ignoring the prehospital history
- Not pursuing an adequate differential diagnosis
- Poor discharge planning

DOCUMENTATION SKILLS

One basic skill that an emergency physician must master is that of superior charting practice. It is well recognized that the medical record is the first line of defense in any claim brought forth, and that many claims hinge on the written record. Some general concepts are noteworthy:

- Remember that what is not on the chart 'did not happen'
- Address all abnormal tests
- Perform interval progress notes
- Read the nurses notes; correct if necessary
- Chart conversations with physicians and consultants
- Time your entries
- Never retrospectively alter a medical record

SPECIFIC HIGH RISK CLINICAL SYNDROMES

Myocardial Infarction

There are more than five million patients per year who present to emergency departments with chest pain as a primary or secondary complaint. Sorting out these cases is difficult as they include a very heterogeneous group of patients, with sources of pain that include cardiac illness, respiratory problems and gastrointestinal illness.

Approximately 1.25 million acute myocardial infarctions occur each year in the United States. This translates into a range of 12,500-50,000 cases of missed MI per year. Settlement figures for typical cases are on the order of about $250-300,000.

There have been numerous modern advances in medical technology, and multiple technologies to assist clinicians in the diagnosis of acute myocardial infarction (AMI). Among these are sophisticated enzyme markers, stress thallium tests, echocardiography. Despite these new aids in detection, numerous studies reveal that emergency physicians still misdiagnose and discharge between 2-8% of acute myocardial infarctions from the primary care setting.

Clearly, this is a category in which clinicians focus if they want to make headway into the litigation landscape of emergency medicine. Some common recurring themes in cases involving AMI include:

- Missed EKG changes
- Failure to note serial EKG changes over time
- Failure to obtain old EKG's for comparison
- Ignoring non specific ST-T changes.
- Failure to obtain and record a good history
- Failure to recognize the importance of prior cardiac disease
- Failure to appreciate the atypical presentation

- Using inappropriate bedside diagnostic techniques (GI cocktails to make a diagnosis)

By developing a robust knowledge base in emergency cardiac concepts, emergency physicians can be prepared to properly treat this very high risk aspect of acute care in the ED.

The Febrile Child

The evaluation of children who present to the emergency department with fever remains a high risk scenario for physicians. Because the damages in these cases are often so catastrophic, the settlements and awards are often in the multi-million dollar range. In the American College of Emergency Physicians (ACEP) closed claims study, while pediatric meningitis cases accounted for only 2.3% of cases filed, it led to over 15% of total settlement and award dollars paid out.

Fortunately, the development of H. Influenza vaccine has led to a decline in the incidence of meningitis since the late 1980s. In immunized children the incidence has declined by more than 90%, and through "herd immunity", by more than 70% in unimmunized children. Nevertheless, diagnosing meningitis in children continues to be problematic, and remains a cause for anxiety among emergency physicians.

For febrile children with an apparent central nervous system (CNS) focus of infection, and especially when there are documented terms by nursing staff describing the child with key trigger terms, such as "irritable", "lethargic", "inconsolable", "not feeding", etc., it is incumbent on the physician to initiate a full febrile workup, including cultures and lumbar puncture.

On the other hand, for febrile children with no CNS source of infection, the physician should go to great lengths to:

- Document is the apparent focus of infection
- Document the lack of clinical evidence of meningitis or toxicity
- Document clinical signs and evidence of wellness on discharge

Infants younger than 6 months of age present a particularly high risk subset in this category of patients. One reason for this is that very young infants frequently do not manifest signs of meningeal irritation, despite evidence of infection in the CNS. With increasing age, infants begin to demonstrate the more classic signs and symptoms associated with meningitis (Table 2).

Table 2: Meningeal Signs vs. Age

Age	Meningeal Findings
Less than 6 months of age	27%
6-12 months of age	72%
Greater than 12 months of age	93%

The precise age at which to perform a full septic workup in neonates remains controversial, but most authorities recommend conservative management for children less than 2 months of age.

If sepsis or meningitis is in fact diagnosed in a child, the next most paramount action the emergency physician must take is the initiation of treatment for the condition. This sounds intuitive, but many lawsuits result from a delay in treatment for meningitis or sepsis. Talan, et al, studied the time from registration in the emergency department to antibiotic administration, and found the mean to be 2.7 hours. Meadow, et al, performed a similar study in two separate hospitals, and found a mean time of administration to be 2.70 and 2.79 hours. Clearly, physicians are on average, far afield from the published standards which mandate antibiotic administration within 30-60 minutes.

General Risk management suggestions for the evaluation of febrile children can be summarized as follows:

- In this scenario, perhaps more than any other, be sure to spend adequate time with the patient and the family
- Watch for "trigger" terms on the nursing notes
- Document your findings in great detail
- Document the wellness of the child on discharge
- Avoid relying too much on lab tests ("normal" CBC) or on the apparent response to antipyretics
- Be sure you have arranged for rigorous close follow up

Wounds

In contrast to some other entities, wounds generally result in a lower mean settlement amount, but occur with a much higher frequency. In the ACEP closed claims study, wounds resulted in less than 10% of the total dollars paid out, yet represented over 27% of the total number of cases brought.

The cases tend to involve a select few recurrent themes or categories. These include:

- Failure to diagnose retained foreign bodies
- Failure to diagnose tendon injuries
- Failure to diagnose nerve injuries
- Failure to diagnose compartment syndromes
- Inadequate management of animal or human bit injuries

In these cases, the "performance gap" which clinicians are often guilty of, involves some common fact patterns:

- Mistaken reliance on seemingly normal tendon function, without full direct visualization of the tendon
- Inadequate examination of the wound to see foreign bodies or injuries to deep structures

- Ignoring histories which should trigger suspicion of foreign bodies and/or deep structure injuries
- Inadequate use of radiography to search for foreign bodies

This is one category of care which emergency physicians can easily improve their risk exposure, even in the absence of new technologies. If prudent proper practice and a high index of suspicion are maintained, the clinician can avoid missing injuries which can result in complications and claims of negligence.

Abdominal Pain-AAA

Abdominal Aortic Aneurysm (AAA) is a subset of the abdominal pain category which plagues emergency physicians as a high risk encounter. It is more widespread than frequently assumed, resulting in 15,000 deaths per year in the United States. Unruptured AAAs exist in an estimated 2-4% of adults, and about 750,000 adults in the U.S. with this entity. Studies suggest that 11% of males older than 65 have an AAA.

It is recognized that AAA can present in many false guises. The classic triad of abdominal pain, decreased blood pressure and pulsatile mass occurred in less than 50% of cases.[15] One study also found that 10% of cases who were referred to urologists for presumed kidney stone actually ended up having a AAA.

However, in addition to these pitfalls, clinicians often perform an inadequate history which might lead to suspecting the diagnosis (e.g. Risk factors such as hypertension or connective tissue disease, history of AAA, family history of AAA).

By obtaining an adequate history, performing a focused physical examination, and by using aggressive imaging studies, a physician will be less likely to be misled to a more attractive but erroneous diagnosis such as diverticulitis or renal colic.

Abdominal Pain- Acute Appendicitis

Acute appendicitis is one of the more common surgical conditions which presents to emergency departments. In addition, failure to diagnose appendicitis is among the more frequent causes of malpractice litigation. The ACEP study found almost 5% of litigation dollars paid out were for failure to diagnose appendicitis. As many as 30% of patients who ultimately prove to have appendicitis have been previously seen at least once and discharged by another physician.

Appendicitis is often missed on initial presentation because it frequently simulates other disease entities such as gastroenteritis and pelvic inflammatory disease. The frequent aberrant position of the appendix relative to the cecum makes the symptoms of appendicitis variable in location and nature, which contributes to the difficulty in diagnosis.

Sometimes, a patient presents very early in the course of the disease, at which time it may literally be impossible to make the diagnosis. An early presentation may evolve over such a long period of time that the diagnosis does not become clear even after a reasonable observation period in the emergency department. In these situations, it is imperative for the clinician to arrange for close follow up and reassessment, either by the patient's primary care physician, or even back in the emergency department where the original evaluation took place.

This category is one in which, perhaps more than any other category discussed, it behooves the physician to engage in detailed dialogue with the patient and their family. In this way, the priorities for evaluation can be communicated, and reasonable patient expectations can be established. A patient who understands the limitations of evaluating undifferentiated abdominal pain, and the potential possibilities, will be less likely to be angry if there is an unexpected diagnosis or untoward outcome.

Subarachnoid Hemorrhage

Headache is one of the more frequent presenting complaints to emergency departments. Many of these result from more benign causes, such as tension or migraine headaches. Unfortunately, a subset are caused by subarachnoid hemorrhage (SAH), which can be catastrophic, particularly if not diagnosed early.

Research indicates that about 10-15 million citizens in the United States harbor intracranial aneurysms. Every year, approximately 30,000 people sustain a nontraumatic SAH from these aneurysms or from other arterial-venous malformations in the CNS. The peak age is around 55-60 years of age, but 20% occur between15-45 years of age.

Some studies reveal that over half of cases of SAH are missed during the initial medical evaluation for headache. One reason for this seemingly high misdiagnosis rate is that while headache is a frequent presenting complaint, the incidence of SAH is relatively low relative to the overall number of total cases of headache. Sentinel bleeds which can sometimes can present a clue to the correct diagnosis can be subtle and present with a varying array of symptoms that can confuse even the most astute clinician.

Litigation cases involving SAH frequently reveal that the clinician failed to have an adequate index of suspicion relative to the presenting history. Poor risk analysis and poor documentation of history and physical findings are often noted in these cases. In patients presenting with headache, a detailed neurological exam is imperative to perform and document. Aggressive use of neuroimaging studies and a liberal use lumbar puncture must be the standard practice for clinicians if they want to avoid missing this diagnosis.

MISCELLANEOUS RISK ENTITIES

Writing Inpatient Orders

It is the expectation or at least historical practice of some hospitals to have the emergency physician write initial "holding" orders on patients whom they admit to primary care physicians. This practice is to be discouraged. It extends the liability of the emergency physician far beyond the scope of the patient's original care in the emergency department.

It may be necessary for the emergency department director to vigorously lobby the medical staff and the administrators of their institution to achieve the abandonment of this practice. ACEP has published a position paper stating it does not condone this practice.

Patients Who Leave Against Medical Advice

Some patients who present to emergency departments choose for a variety of reasons, to leave either before their evaluation and treatment is complete, or to against the recommendation of the physician who wants to admit them to the hospital.

In these cases, the emergency physician should recognize these scenarios as high risk situations, since the presenting complaint has likely not been fully assessed. The clinician should try to work out whatever issue the patient may have to avert the departure. Often the patient has a relatively minor issue or problem that is causing them to consider departure. If these can be corrected, the situation can often be defused, and the original plan of evaluation, treatment, or admission can continue.

However, even after taking these steps, some patients still will continue with their intention to leave the department. In this case, detailed documentation by the emergency physician again becomes critical. The physician should document clearly:

- That the patient has expressed a desire to leave
- That this departure is against the judgment and advice of the physician
- That the patient has been informed of the risks and potential consequences of such an action
- That the patient understands these risks and potential outcomes, and still chooses to leave

Case law review in the U.S. reveals that if these principles are followed, this imparts a very protective effect for the physician. Certainly, the patient must be judged to be competent to make such a decision. The patient's competence should be noted, and that it is an informed decision the patient is making.

Transfers

A surprising number of medicolegal cases involve the transfer of patients from one facility to another. This activity is one that is underappreciated as a high risk situation by emergency physicians, even when done appropriately and correctly. It is fraught with even more peril when done improperly.

The burden is on the transferring physician to ascertain that the patient is stable for transfer. One guiding principle is that the monitoring and treatment capabilities must always be maintained before, during, and after the transfer is complete.

This means that a critically ill patient who in the emergency department has EKG monitoring in place and access to endotracheal intubation should it become necessary, should not be transferred in a vehicle which does not have this equipment or with personnel not capable of performing these interventions. In these cases, a basic life support crew of emergency medical technicians would not be appropriate to use for such a transfer, because this would constitute a "downgrade" of monitoring and treatment capability for that patient.

Proper protocol dictates that the receiving physician must accept transfer of the patient in question. In addition, the patient themselves must provide a written consent to the transfer, after being informed of the reason for transfer. This informed consent should be documented on the medical record, ideally on a form designed to cover the requisite elements recommended for transfer of patients to other institutions.

OTHER TOOLS TO LESSEN RISK

In addition to personal professional practice habits, there are other tools that are an important part of an overall program to control and lessen the medicolegal risk of emergency departments. These include:

- A Functioning quality Assurance Program
- An X-ray/EKG/Lab over read system
- A telephone callback system for high risk cases
- A complaint management program
- Periodic physician education on the tenets and principles of risk management

With these practices and with a coordinated departmental effort, the risk for individual clinicians, as well as for the emergency department and its parent institution can be reduced. Having achieved this, they can more readily accomplish their primary mission of bringing high quality care to their patients.

REFERENCES

1. Rogers, JT: Risk Management in Emergency Medicine. American College of Emergency Physicians publication; 1985:4-5.
2. Karcz A, et al: Preventability of malpractice claims in emergency medicine: a closed claims study. Ann Emerg Med 1993; 22:553-559.
3. Selker HP: Coronary care unit triage decision aids: how do we know when they work? Am J Med. 1989;87:491-493.
4. Braunwald E, Mark DB, et al: Unstable angina: diagnosis and management. Clinical practice guideline number 10. Rockville, MD: Agency for Health Care Policy and Research and the National Heart, Lung, and Blood Institute, Public Health Service, U.S. Dept. of Health and Human Services. 1994: 154.
5. National Heart, Lung and Blood Institute: Morbidity and Mortality Chartbook on Cardiovascular, Lung, and Blood Disease. Bethesda, MD: National Institutes of Health, 1994, U.S. Dep. of Health and Human Services.
6. Lee, TH, Rouan, GW, et al: Clinical characteristics and history of patients sent home from the emergency room. Am J Cardiol 1987; 60:220-224.

7. McCarthy BD, Beshansky, JR, et al: Missed diagnoses of acute MI in the emergency room. Results of a multicenter study. Ann Emerg Med 1993; 22:579.

8. Adams WG, et al: Decline in childhood Hemophilus influenza in the Hib vaccine era. JAMA. 1993;269:221-226.

9. Trautlein JJ, et al: Malpractice in the emergency department- review of 200 cases. Ann Emerg Med. 1984; 13:709-711.

10. Walsh-Kelly C. et al: Clinical predictors of bacterial versus aseptic meningitis in childhood. Ann Emerg Med 1992;21:910:914.

11. Rothrock SG, et al: The febrile child: assessment, risk reduction, and general principles of emergency management. Emergency Medicine Reports. 1995;16:193-9.

12. Talan, DA, et al: Relationship of clinical presentation to time of antibiotics for emergency department management of suspected bacterial meningitis. Ann Emerg Med. 1993;22:1733-1738.

13. Meadow, et al: Ought 'standard of care' be the 'standard of care'?: A study of the time it takes to administer antibiotics to children with meningitis. AJDC 144:428-9.

14. Abdominal Aortic Aneurysm: The case for resection. Circulation: 70: 1.

15. Banerjee A: Atypical manifestations of ruptured abdominal aortic aneurysms. Postgrad Med1993; 69:6-1

16. Role of Ultrasound in detecting AAA in urologic patients. Eur J Vasc Surg. 1993; 7: 298-300.

17. Rothrock, SG, et al: Misdiagnosis of appendicitis in nonpregnanat women of childbearing age. J Emerg Med. 1995; 13:1-8.

18. Rothrock SG: Overcoming the limitations and pitfalls in the diagnosis of appendicitis. Emer Med Reports 1992;13:41-52.

19. Rusnak RA, Borer JM, Fastow JS: Misdiagnosis of appendicitis: common features discovered in cases after litigation. Am J Emerg Med 1994;12:397-402.

20. Mayberg MR, Batjer HH, Day R, et al: Guidelines for the management of SAH: Stroke. 1994;25:2315 -2328.

21. Sacco RL, Wolf PA, Bharucha NE, et al: Subarachnoid and intracranial hemorrhage: Natural history, prognosis, and precursive factors in the Framingham Study. Neurology. 1984; 34: 847-854.

22. Dwyer N, Lang D: "Brain Attack"- SAH-Death due to delayed diagnosis. J Royal College of Physicians London. Vol 31 No. 1 Jan 1997.

23. Adams HP, Jergenson DD, Kassell NF, et al: Pitfalls in the recognition of subarachnoid hemorrhage. JAMA. 1980; 244: 794-796.

EAR, NOSE, AND THROAT EMERGENCIES

Robert Partridge, M.D., M.P.H.[*]

This chapter is a case based approach to common ENT emergencies, including swelling, sore throats, foreign bodies, trauma, epistaxis, and how to manage them.

CASE ONE: ADULT EPIGLOTTITIS

A 25 year old man presents with drooling, hoarse voice and odynophagia. On physical examination he has a temperature of 38.5 C, and is leaning forward. The oropharynx shows erythematous, symmetrical tonsils, and no exudate. His neck is supple with anterior cervical adenopathy. Adult epiglottitis presents as a sore throat out of proportion to physical findings. All adults with sore throat should have epiglottitis ruled out by the emergency physician. The epiglottis must be directly or indirectly visualized. The emergency physician should be prepared to intervene with endotracheal intubation or cricothyroidotomy. The clinical presentation in adults can be divided in to three categories:

- Category 1 patients have severe respiratory distress and imminent respiratory arrest. Often associated with H. Flu.
- Category 2 patients present with moderate to severe symptoms (can't swallow or lie down) and signs (muffled voice, stridor, accessory muscle use) of airway compromise.
- Category 3 patients have mild to moderate respiratory distress, and the progression of their illness is usually longer, ranging from 3-14 days.

Category 1 and 2 patients usually require definitive airway management in the emergency department or in the operating room. However, most adults are category 3, and can be safely observed in the intensive care unit without intubation or other airway

[*] Robert Partridge, M.D., M.P.H., Assistant Professor of Medicine, Brown Medical School, Department of Emergency Medicine, Rhode Island Hospital, Providence, Rhode Island

intervention. All patients with epiglottitis are treated antibiotics to cover staph, strep, and H. influenza. Ideal antibiotics include ceftriaxone, cefuroxime and ampicillin/sulbactam. There is little evidence to support the use of steroids in epiglottitis. Heliox as an adjunct can be used to gain some time for the patient with severe respiratory distress while preparations are made for intubation or a surgical airway in the ED or OR.

Failure to consider the diagnosis is the most common error made in the evaluation if epiglottis. Airway management should be done by an experienced physician. Nasal intubation is contraindicated in epiglottitis. The possibility of sudden airway obstruction should always be considered, and all patients require close monitoring.

CASE TWO: ANGIOEDEMA

A 48 year old woman with a history of hypertension presents with a 1 day history of progressive tongue swelling. She takes an angiotensin converting enzyme inhibitor daily. Angioedema can be divided into hereditary and acquired types. Hereditary angioedema is an inherited deficiency of the inhibitor of the first activated component of complement. The more common acquired angioedema occurs in association with allergens (food, drugs). ACE inhibitors are a common cause, and can occur months or years after initiating therapy. Treatment of this condition requires careful attention to the airway as angioedema can occasionally progress to complete airway obstruction, and oral endotracheal intubation may be impossible. Standard treatment includes H1 blockers, steroids and epinephrine, although these may be less effective in hereditary angioedema. In such patients, C1 inhibitor concentrates may be required. If pharmacologic intervention is ineffective and patients progress to respiratory distress, nasotracheal intubation may be the easiest way to establish an airway. Patients with angioedema can usually be observed in the ED for several hours and if symptoms are resolving they can usually be discharged home. Patients with no improvement or at risk for respiratory compromise should be admitted to the ICU and preparations should be made for stabilization of the airway.

CASE THREE: NASAL FOREIGN BODY

Nasal foreign bodies are common problems in the 2-4 year old age group. Patients will usually present in one of two ways. Either they will have been observed by their caretaker to have put something in to their nose, or they may have unilateral pain, bleeding, discharge, odor, sneezing or fever. Any object that is small enough to fit in the nares may be found, but of all common objects, button batteries are particularly worrisome because they can cause local tissue necrosis. In the differential diagnosis of a patient with symptoms of nasal foreign body would be simple sinusitis, tumor or epistaxis unrelated to the foreign body. The evaluation of a patient with a known or suspected foreign body includes determining the type of foreign body, time of insertion and symptoms since insertion. The examination should only be done only after all equipment has been assembled. A nasal speculum, headlight, topical vasoconstrictor/anesthetic solution, cotton, bayonet and alligator forceps, suction catheters, #4 Fogarty catheter, right angle hook and ear curette should all be made ready. Assess the patient's cooperativeness. Sedation is usually not necessary. If it is not clear which nostril contains the foreign body, use a mirror held under the nose. The obstructed nostril will not fog the mirror with expiration. Sinuses should be percussed and illuminated. If the foreign body is not visible on initial inspection, prepare the nasal mucosa with 4% cocaine before deeper inspection. Nasal x-rays and facial CT scan may also be useful in determining the site and type of foreign body.

How do you get them out? First, have the patient blow their nose, or have the child's parent blow forcefully into the child's mouth (a mouth to mouth maneuver) in an attempt to force out the foreign body. If instruments are required, flat objects can usually be removed by alligator forceps and round objects with suction or a Fogarty catheter. Softer materials, such as vegetable or wood matter should be removed with a minimum of manipulation. Disc batteries should be removed without being crushed and without causing bleeding, with can increase the chance of tissue necrosis. A right angle hook is often useful in removing disc batteries. Complications associated with foreign body removal include aspiration, sinusitis and epistaxis. An ENT consultant should be called for a disc battery that cannot be removed, aspiration, or infection. The most likely error the emergency physician is likely to make with nasal foreign bodies is a missed foreign body due to failure to consider the diagnosis or a poor exam.

CASE FOUR: PERICHONDRITIS

Perichondritis is an infection of the fibrous connective tissue surrounding the cartilaginous external ear. It can occur following burns, trauma, chemical injury, otitis externa, or a furuncle of the canal. This infection is usually caused by staph, strep or pseudomonas. Perichondritis can be distinguished clinically from chondritis because chondritis causes auricular deformity; in perichondritis, the external architecture of the ear is preserved. Perichondritis is treated with local cleansing, a combination antibiotic and steroid cream, and an oral fluoroquinolone. Left untreated, perichondritis can lead to necrosis of the cartilage of the external ear, resulting in deformity. Patients with perichondritis can be managed by the emergency physician, and referred to ENT for follow up.

CASE FIVE: EPISTAXIS

Emergency physicians are often manage patients with epistaxis. Epistaxis is characterized clinically by active bleeding from one or both nares and/or the posterior nasopharynx. Retrograde flow may occur into the orbit via the lacrimal duct. Patients are often hypertensive, but blood pressure may be labile, and shock may occur. Epistaxis can occur as a result of trauma, mucosal drying, topical vasoconstrictors, foreign bodies, forceful blowing, surgery and neoplasms. Hypertension and coagulopathies do not cause epistaxis. Epistaxis can be classified as anterior (site can be visualized by examiner) and posterior (site cannot be visualized). Over 90% of bleeds are anterior, usually located in the heavily vascularized area of Kiesselbach's plexus on the nasal septum. Almost all epistaxis can be managed by the emergency physician.

The initial evaluation includes ABC's and vital signs. In the stable patient, the next step is preparation for rhinoscopy. The emergency physician must identify the site of bleeding to effective manage epistaxis. The examiner should be gowned and gloved and the patient gowned. The examiner should also use a mask for face and eye protection. Any clots should be evacuated by blowing or suction, and the soft part of the nose pinched for 10 minutes. During this time, additional history can be obtained including trauma, medications, previous episodes, and hepatic or systemic disease. Time of onset and which nare bled first should also be elicited. The nare that bled first likely contains the site of bleeding. Laboratory testing, specifically for CBC and coagulation studies may be obtained. Cardiac monitoring, pulse oximetry, and IV fluids should be initiated on hemodynamically unstable patients and the elderly. Patients should be positioned upright and leaning forward. Anterior rhinoscopy should then be performed, using a nasal speculum and a light source.

If the site of bleeding is found (sometimes it may be necessary to make a patient re-bleed to correctly identify the site), apply a topical vasoconstrictors and anesthetic. Cocaine 4%, tetracaine 4% with epinephrine (1:1000) mixed 1:1, or phenylephrine 0.25% may be used. These medicines can be soaked in cotton pledgets and placed in the nares for 10 minutes. Cautery of the bleeding site can be achieved with silver nitrate applicators, which should be rolled over the area surrounding the bleeding site. There must be some moisture present for them to work. Care should be taken not to maintain pressure on one particular area of the septum or on both sides of the septum as necrosis of the cartilage may result. Topical absorbable hemostatic agents may also be used to cauterize anterior bleeds. Local injection of lidocaine 1% and epinephrine (1:100,000) is another alternative for control of anterior bleeds.

If the above measures fail, anterior nasal packing should be performed, either using a traditional petrolatum gauze or a compressed surgical sponge nasal tampon. Gauze packing can be difficult for the novice and requires good initial anesthesia. Compressed surgical sponges should be trimmed, lubricated, pushed straight back into position in the nostril, and then wetted so that it expands into place.

Posterior packs should be used if the site of bleeding cannot be visualized or if an anterior pack fails. Traditional posterior packs with rolled gauze are uncomfortable for the patient and require time and skill on the part of the physician. Easier posterior packs can be achieved using devices with inflatable anterior and posterior balloons or by using a 16Fr. foley catheter with a 30cc balloon. An anterior pack should always be placed after a posterior packing has been applied. Posterior packs carry an increased risk of complication, including hypoventilation, hypoxia, hypercarbia, dysphagia and arrhythmias, and for these reasons patients with posterior packs should be admitted. Finally, if a posterior pack is not effective, arterial ligation or endoscopic cautery under direct vision may be attempted by the ENT surgeon. Alternately, selective arterial embolization can be done by an interventional radiologist.

Patients with epistaxis are often hypertensive, however this almost always resolves when the epistaxis has been controlled. In general, treat the epistaxis first and you won't have to worry about the hypertension. Prophylactic antibiotics should be given to all patients with anterior and posterior packs. Admit all patients with posterior packs, extensive blood loss or those with co-morbid disease (frail, elderly or COPD). Remember – prepare adequately, identify the bleeding site properly, and consider foreign body in all children with epistaxis as epistaxis is uncommon in children.

CASE SIX: PEDIATRIC EPIGLOTTITIS

A 4 year old child presents with acute onset of fever, drooling and stridor. She complained of sore throat earlier that morning. She has received no immunizations. On physical exam she has a temperature of 39.4 C, pulse 128, respirations 32 and BP 114/72. She has inspiratory stridor and is in acute distress. She will not permit and examination of the oropharynx, and is sitting up, mouth open, chin forward and drooling.

The differential diagnosis in this case would include epiglottitis, viral croup, retropharyngeal abscess, peritonsillar abscess (rare under age 10) and diptheria. This patient has the 4 "D's" of epiglottitis – dysphagia, dysphonia, drooling and distress. Epiglottitis is the swelling of the supraglottic structures at the hyoid level, and is usually caused by HIB, staph, beta-hemolytic strep, M. Catarrhalis and pneumococcus. It is an acute respiratory emergency and all children with epiglottitis should have their airway secured with endotracheal intubation. Children should be transported directly to the OR for this procedure. They should not be distressed in advance by attempting venipuncture or other invasive procedures. If the diagnosis of epiglottitis is in question, it is permissible for the stable child to have a lateral radiograph of the neck (with a physician skilled in airway management at the bedside at all times), to confirm or exclude the diagnosis. If respiratory arrest occurs, attempt ventilation with an ambu-bag prior to attempting intubation. Use a small endotracheal tube and a stylet. If intubation is impossible, needle cricothyroidotomy with a 14 gauge IV catheter over needle directed caudad should be attempted. All children with epiglottitis should be admitted to intensive care and given antibiotics – cefuroxime, ceftriaxone, cefotaxime or choramphenicol are recommended.

CASE SEVEN: RETROPHARYNGEAL ABSCESS

A 7 year old child presents with fever, neck pain and sore throat. He is in no respiratory distress, and a soft tissue neck radiograph shows marked swelling of the retropharyngeal tissues. Retropharyngeal abscess is usually seen in children, often as a result of infection of the lymph nodes in the retropharyngeal space. This disease can occur in adults due to ingested foreign bodies (e.g. fish bones) or trauma to the posterior pharyngeal wall. These infections are frequently polymicrobial, with staph, strep and anerobes most commonly cultured.

Clinically patients present with fever, neck pain and sore throat out of proportion to oropharyngeal findings. They may have odynophasia, neck swelling, drooling and stridor. The voice may be muffled if the swelling is above the larynx, but will be normal if the swelling is below the larynx. Patients appear toxic, dehydrated, pale, and the head is held stiff. Chest pain suggests mediastinal extension ,which can occur by direct extension through fascial planes. ED evaluation and management includes airway assessment and monitoring, CT scan of the neck and chest, IV fluids, IV antibiotics and ENT surgeon consult for incision and drainage in the OR.

CASE EIGHT: SUBMANDIBULAR ABSCESS

A 68 year old woman presents with a 3 day history of fever, pain and swelling under the tongue. On physical examination, pus can be seen draining from Wharton's duct. Submandibular abscess, often the result of a duct obstruction by a stone is often the precursor to Ludwig's angina, which can cause rapid airway compromise. The role or the emergency physician is first airway assessment, and then to determine the extent of the involvement of 3 contiguous spaces in the mandible - the submandibular space, the submental space, and the sublingual space. This may be possible clinically, but if not CT scan should be performed. Involvement of all three spaces is Ludwig's angina, and the patient should be prepared for the OR. If aggressive airway intervention is needed, nasotracheal intubation is preferred as massive submandibular swelling precludes orotracheal intubation. All patients require IV antibiotics with ampicillin/sulbactam, clindamycin, or 2nd/ 3rd generation cephalosporins to cover strep and other oral flora. The ENT surgeon should be consulted for incision and drainage. If the abscess involves only one of the submandibular, submental or sublingual spaces, and is well localized, the patient can be discharged home with close ENT follow up. All other patients should be admitted.

CASE NINE: TONGUE LACERATION

Tongue lacerations are common in children, and frequently occur as a result of a fall. Tongue lacerations can be managed by the emergency physician without the need for subspecialty intervention. Only certain lacerations require repair – those involving the edge, lacerations passing completely through the tongue, large flaps or persistent bleeding. Small flaps on the edge should be revised. Smaller, superficial lacerations do not require repair. Repair is achieved by first anesthetizing the tongue with 4% lidocaine soaked in gauze applied directly to the tongue for 5 minutes. Conscious sedation is needed for larger lacerations or less cooperative patients. Silk or absorbable suture should be used for closure, and all 3 layers (inferior mucosa, muscle and superior mucosa) should be closed.

CASE TEN: LINGUAL TONSILLITIS

A 25 year old female complains of 2 days of sore throat, then suddenly develops 2 hours of progressive difficulty and stridor. On examination only diffuse inflammation is seen in the oropharynx, and fever and leukocytosis are often present. The diagnosis is made on lateral soft tissue radiograph. Lingual tonsillitis usually occurs in an adult who has previously undergone pallatine tonsillectomy. Treatment is to first secure the airway, which often requires cricothyroidotomy or emergent tracheotomy. Intravenous fluids and antibiotics should be administered, and the patient admitted after ENT consultation.

CASE ELEVEN: BLOWOUT FRACTURE OF THE ORBIT

An 18 year old man presents stating he was punched in the right eye the night before. He did not lose consciousness and has normal vital signs. His visual acuity (part of the exam for blowout fracture which must be done) is 20/40 OD, and 20/20 OS. He has decreased extraocular motion both superiorly and laterally, but pupils are equal and reactive, and ocular pressures are equal. Slit lamp examination is normal. A blowout fracture of the orbit occurs when force into the anterior orbit is transmitted to the orbital floor. Clinical features include lid edema, chemosis, subconjunctival hemorrhage, infraorbital anesthesia, enopthalmos diplopia and lower pupillary level on the affected side. Blowout fractures require careful evaluation early on to exclude an ocular injury. If exam is delayed, eyelid swelling can make ocular evaluation extremely difficult. Look for corneal abrasions, hyphema, ruptured globe, vitreous bleed or retinal detachment. Surgical consultation by the ENT or plastic surgeon is required for enopthalmos, hypopthalmos or muscular entrapment. Surgical intervention is contraindicated if there is concurrent hyphema, retinal tear, globe perforation or a single eye.

CASE TWELVE: DENTAL FRACTURE

A 22 year old male chipped his tooth while playing football. He complains of severe pain and heat/cold sensitivity. Tooth fractures are described using the Ellis classification. Ellis class I fractures involve the enamel, and aside from cosmetics are asymptomatic for the patient. Ellis class II fractures involve the dentin, a porous tissue, that results in heat and cold sensitivity and increases susceptibility to nerve necrosis and abscess. Ellis class III fractures extend into the pulp (nerve), which also results in extreme heat and cold sensitivity as well as risk of abscess. A root canal is required in follow up by the oral surgeon. If a tooth is completely avulsed, it should be reimplanted without being allowed to dry. If this is done within 30 minutes, there is a 90% retention rate. Patients with Ellis II and III fractures should have the affected tooth covered with calcium hydroxide, discharged with analgesics, and referred for root canal.

CASE THIRTEEN: SEPTIC NASAL SEPTAL HEMATOMA

A 48 year old male presents 3 days after being involved in a fight. He complains of nasal pain and fever. A nasal septal hematoma occurs after trauma as the perichondrium surrounding the nasal septum is separated from the cartilage. The result is necrosis or abscess of the septal cartilage, meningitis or cavernous sinus thrombosis. Drainage of a septal hematoma should be performed by the emergency physician. This is accomplished by mucosal incision and drainage, or aspiration with an 18 gauge needle. An anterior packing is then placed in the nostril. Patients with an uncomplicated septal hematoma can be discharged home with ENT referral. The packing should be removed daily and any recurrent hematoma aspirated. When no new hematoma occurs, the packing can be removed 24 hours later. Patients with complicated hematomas or septic hematomas should be admitted after incision and drainage and started on IV antibiotics.

CASE FOURTEEN: SIALOLITHIASIS

A 44 year old man presents with sudden onset of pain and swelling under the tongue. On examination he has swollen, injected tissue directly under the tongue. The opening of Wharton's duct is inflamed and a small hematoma is present. Sialolithiasis is causes acute obstruction of Wharton's duct and resultant swelling of the submandibular salivary gland. Stone formation is favored anatomically as the duct opens upward and sludging can occur. This condition is not always painful, and some patients will experience only painless swelling during salivation. Treatment is to manually remove the stone if it is distal and can be visualized. Prescribe something sour, refer to ENT and place the patient on prophylactic antibiotics.

CASE FIFTEEN: UVULITIS

A 35 year old male presents with 2 days of sore throat, and now states he is choking. On examination, his oropharynx is clear except an enlarged, edematous swollen uvula. Quinke's edema, or uvulitis, occurs as a result of allergic reaction, angioedema, viral illness, bacterial infection (group A strep, H. influenza, S. pneumonia) or trauma. An important distinction for the emergency physician to make is whether the uvulitis represents a bacterial infection. The uvula will appear pale in cases of allergic reaction or angioedema, whereas in bacterial uvulitis the uvula will appear erythematous, and may co-exist with pharyngitis or epiglottitis. Treatment is with dexamethasone 10mg IM (frequently used but not proven), antihistamines, gentle saline gargles and topical lidocaine anesthesia to reduce gagging. Suspected bacterial infections should include IV antibiotics and admission. Patients without suspicion for bacterial uvulitis can usually be discharged home.

CASE SIXTEEN: ORAL COMMISURE BURN

A 5 year old male presents after chewing on an electrical cord. On examination he has second and third degree burns bilaterally to the oral commisures. There is no bleeding. Oral commisure burns may initially appear localized only to extend over the following 3-5 days. Bleeding will occur 7-10 days after injury, heralded by a bloody ooze around the eschar. Massive delayed bleeding will then occur from the labial artery, as the eschar sloughs off. The important thing for the emergency physician to realize is that massive delayed bleeding will occur. Management can be done in one of two ways. Either the patient can be admitted and observed until surgical repair can be done by the ENT or plastic surgeon, or the patient can be admitted on post injury day 4 for delayed primary excision and closure. The risk of delayed bleeding is increased in younger children.

REFERENCES

1. Harwood-Nuss, *A. The Clinical Practactice of Emergency Medicine*, 3rd Ed.. Lippincott, Williams and Wilkins, Philadelphia, 2001.

2. Rosen, Barkin, Eds. *Emergency Medicine*, 4th Ed. Mosby, 1998.
3. Roberts, Hedges. Clinical *Procedures in Emergency Medicine,* 3rd Ed. W.B.Saunders Company, Philadelphia, 1998.

BIOTERRORISM

Robert Partridge, M.D., M.P.H.[*]

Biological terrorism is the intentional release of biological agents into the environment to cause disease or death in a population. The recent anthrax cases in the United States have demonstrated that bioterrorism is a real threat for civilian populations, and that emergency medicine is the first line of defense against any biological attack. Practitioners of emergency medicine need to be prepared for a bioterrorism event, equipped to identify and detect and event, as well as evaluate and treat persons who may have been exposed to biological agents. Emergency medicine practitioners should be familiar with the likely agents that might be used in a bioterrorism event.

The first issue to address is why biological agents would be directed against any population by any person or group. The simple answer is because these agents, if delivered successfully have the potential to cause catastrophic morbidity and mortality in almost any population. Biological agents may have devastating effects even though only small amounts are required. These agents are usually invisible, odorless, tasteless, easy to obtain and difficult to detect. Civilian populations are generally unprotected, the onset of symptoms is delayed, and the agents are difficult to trace. In addition to devastating morbidity and mortality, any bioterrorism event can be crippling to a nation because fear and chaos could cause the "worried well" to overwhelm the health care infrastructure.

Why be prepared? Biological terrorism is not new. Centuries ago, cadavers were used to contaminate enemy water supplies, and the intentional introduction of smallpox into virgin populations has been well documented. In the modern world, arsenals of military bioweapons exist that have been engineered for mass dissemination as aerosols. Terrorists, who may even be "homegrown", may have access to these agents. Many of these agents are highly contagious and fatal, and populations worldwide are susceptible. In addition, biological agents do not stop at political boundaries, and some, such as smallpox can be quickly spread worldwide by passengers on commercial airliners.

It has been postulated that the most likely scenario for a biological terrorism event in the US would be an aerosol release in a major city, or at a large event or key function.

---

[*] Robert Partridge, M.D., M.P.H., Assistant Professor of Medicine, Brown Medical School, Department of Emergency Medicine, Rhode Island Hospital, Providence, Rhode Island

The onset of symptoms would be delayed so that victims would likely present to different emergency departments or their doctors' offices. As the number of affected people increased and an event was identified, local emergency departments would be overwhelmed with patients and resources would be exhausted. Recognition of initial exposure would be determined using epidemiologic methods. The Centers for Disease Control has estimated that an aerosolized release of 100 kg of anthrax spores upwind of Washington, D.C. in the right atmospheric conditions would result in 130,000- 3 million deaths, and cost an estimated $26.2 billion per 100,000 persons exposed.

Large scale outbreaks will require rapid mobilization of public health workers, emergency responders and private health care providers, as well as rapid procurement of drugs and vaccines. The initial detection of a covert biological attack will occur at the local level – in hospital emergency departments, doctors' offices and clinics. Only a short time will elapse between identification of the first cases and the second wave of population illness. Mixed in with those exposed will be a larger group of "worried well" who may have many non-specific symptoms, but no disease. Early detection is critical for ensuring prompt and effective treatment for those actually exposed. The challenge for emergency physicians is to identify those who are ill or who have been exposed from the larger group who present for evaluation. In the event of an attack, the local and national health infrastructure could be overwhelmed with large numbers of patients. Medical supplies, diagnostic tests and hospital beds would be inadequate. In addition, emergency medical services workers, hospital employees and public health officials would be at special risk.

The initial detection of a biological attack will be made by primary care providers, with the assistance of local health departments, national health departments (e.g. CDC or National Health Service), disease surveillance systems and epidemiologists. These organizations or specialists can help determine whether an event was a naturally occurring event or an intentional release, can assist in the identification of the pathogen, and can assist with treatment protocols.

There are numerous indicators of a biological attack. Groups of individuals who become ill simultaneously, a sudden increase in illness of healthy people or a sudden increase in non-specific illnesses (e.g. gastrointestinal illnesses) may indicate a biological exposure. An aerosol attack would be suggested by an increase in respiratory presentations of disease. Simultaneous outbreaks in human and animal populations, clusters of rare or unexplained illnesses (e.g. anthrax, brucellosis, eastern equine encephalitis), or disease outside of its normal geographic area are also indicators of an attack. Other indicators include outbreak of disease in an area without a vector or multi-drug resistant pathogens.

The recent anthrax exposures are not the only bioterrorism event in the US in modern history. An intentional biological exposure occurred in The Dalles, Oregon in 1984 by followers of the Rajneeshee cult, who contaminated salad bars at 10 local restaurants with Salmonella. This was done in an attempt to influence local election outcomes and resulted in 751 Salmonella cases. This event was confirmed 18 months after the incident when it was epidemiologically determined that there was no common link between the 10 restaurants, and a member of the cult confessed to the event.

Public health agencies must also be prepared for biological attack. National public health agencies must enhance their capacity to detect and respond to biological attacks, and supply diagnostic reagents to regional public health agencies. Communication programs must be established so that various health agencies can exchange information and to educate and update providers. Public health agencies should also be responsible for enhancing bioterrorism related education and training for health care professionals, and prepare educational materials to inform the public. In addition, public health agencies must stockpile appropriate drugs and vaccines, establish surveillance programs to track microbial strains, support development of diagnostic tests and encourage research on antiviral drugs and vaccines.

The CDC has identified 3 categories of agents that would likely be used in a biological attack. The *highest priority agents* are those that can be easily disseminated from person to person, cause high mortality, have a potential for a major public health impact, are capable of causing widespread panic and social disruption, and require special action for public health preparedness. These highest priority agents include Variola major (smallpox), Bacillus anthracis (anthrax), Yersinia pestis (plague), Clostridium botulinum toxin (botulism), Francisella tularensis (tularemia), filoviruses (Lassa, Junin). Almost all of these agents have been weaponized in the past by various governments. *The second highest priority agents* are those that are moderately easy to disseminate, cause moderate morbidity and low mortality, and still require enhanced diagnostic capacity and surveillance. Second highest priority agents include Coxiella burnetti (Q fever), Brucella species (brucellosis), Burkholderia species (glanders), alphaviruses (encephalitides), ricin toxin from ricinus communis (castor beans). Clostridium perferingens toxins, Staphylococcus enterotoxin B, salmonella species, shigella dysenteriae, escherichia coli 0157:H7, Vibrio cholerae and Cryptosporidium parvum. The *third highest priority agents* include emerging pathogens that could be easily engineered for mass dissemination in the future because of availability, ease of production and dissemination, and potential for high morbidity and mortality and a major public health impact. These agents include Nipah virus, hantaviruses, tickborne hemorrhagic fever viruses, tickborne encephalitis viruses, yellow fever and multi-drug resistant tuberculosis.

SMALLPOX

Spread by respiratory route
Symptoms: malaise, fever, rigors, vomiting, headache, systemic toxicity. 2-3 days later, centripetal rash
Incubation period 10-12 days.
30% mortality (unvaccinated)
Diagnosis: specialized lab
Isolation: respiratory – strict quarantine for 17 days
Treatment: supportive; vaccine available (effective if given to contacts within 3-4 days); immune globulin; antivirals may be effective

ANTHRAX

Agent: Bacillus anthracis, a Gm + spore forming organism
Disease: Skin, oral, respiratory
Presentation: Latency up to 60 days, incubation period 1-5 days.
Symptoms: Fever, malaise, dry cough, chest tightness initially, then slight improvement, followed by severe respiratory distress, septic shock and hemorrhagic mediastinitis. On CXR widened mediastinum and pleural effusions. Death comes in 24-36 hours. Mortality 80-90% untreated. Cutaneous anthrax manifests with a pruritic macule that changes into a painless black eschar. Antibiotic therapy decreases the risk of systemic disease. Mortality untreated is 5-20%
Diagnosis: ELISA to detect toxin
Isolation: Standard
Treatment: Less effective once symptoms have started; ciprofloxacin, doxycycline, or penicillin + streptomycin for 60 days.
Prophylaxis: Vaccine available

In the US in the fall of 2001, anthrax contaminated letters were sent through the postal system. 19 cases of anthrax were confirmed on the east coast, 11 inhalational, 8 cutaneous. All but 2 cases of inhalational anthrax occurred in postal workers. Almost 20,000 postal workers in New York, New Jersey and Washington, DC were offered ciprofloxacin prophylaxis for 60 days. Lessons learned from this event: 1) exposure determines the need for prophylaxis, 2) the use of 2 or more antimicrobials may be useful in treating inhalational anthrax, 3) mass prophylaxis of potentially exposed persons may be effective, and 4) postal sorting machines effectively aerosolize anthrax spores. During this event anyone felt to be potentially exposed to anthrax were referred to local emergency departments for evaluation.

PLAGUE

Agent: Yersinia Pestis, a gram negative bacillus
Exposure: respiratory or vector route
Presentation: incubation period 1-3 days, presents as bubonic, pneumonic or primary septicemic disease. Pneumonic felt to be most likely in a biological attack
Symptoms: malaise, fever, chills, headache, myalgia, cough with hemoptysis. Progresses to fulminant pneumonia, bloody sputum, septic shock, ecchymoses, respiratory failure. Untreated mortality for pneumonic plague is 100%.
Diagnosis: Gm stain of blood, sputum, lymph node. ELISA
Isolation: Strict respiratory until treated for 3 days.
Treatment: Streptomycin, doxycycline, chloramphenicol, gentamycin. Usually fatal if treatment not initiated within 24 hours.
Prophylaxis: Vaccine available against bubonic, poor against pneumonic

TULAREMIA

Agent: Francisella Tularensis, an intracellular Gram negative coccobacillus

Exposure: Skin, vector, ingestion, respiratory.
Presentation: Incubation period 2-10 days. Presents as 2 forms: ulceroglandular (skin) and typhoidal (septicemic).
Symptoms: Fever, headache, chills, myalgias, nausea, vomiting, diarrhea. Untreated mortality 35%.
Diagnosis: Culture difficult from blood, sputum, skin. Serology diagnostic (late). Clinical diagnosis difficult due to non-specific symptoms and signs, often no exposure history.
Isolation: Standard
Treatment: Streptomycin, gentamycin, tetracycline, chloramphenicol.
Prophylaxis: Live vaccine available as an investigational drug.

VIRAL HEMORRHAGIC FEVERS

Agents: Ebola, Lassa, Marburg, Sabia, Bolivian HF, Rift Valley Fever (mosquito vector); Congo-Crimean HF (tick vector)
Exposure: Direct contact, vector, respiratory. Highly infectious by aerosol route
Presentation: Incubation period 4-21 days. Fever, myalgias, prostration, petechiae, hemorrhage, shock. Neurologic, pulmonary, hepatic involvement. Mortality up to 90%.
Diagnosis: Viral isolation lab; ELISA, RT-PCR.
Isolation: Contact. Respiratory isolation for pulmonary hemorrhage
Treatment: Supportive; fluids, transfusion, avoid unnecessary procedures. Ribavirin for Lassa, BHF, CCHF, RVF.

Q FEVER

Agent: Coxiella burnetti, a rickettsia-like organism with spore-like form.
Presentation: Incubation period 10-40 days. Low virulence, high infectivity.
Symptoms and signs: Fever, headache, myalgias, malaise, cough. Pulmonary rales common. Low mortality. Malaise may last for months.
Diagnosis: WBC normal, increased liver function tests. Dx confirmed by ELISA or IFA serology.
Isolation: Standard
Treatment: Macrolides, quinalones, trimethoprim/sulfamethoxazole, tetracycline, chloramphenicol. Antibiotics shorten course and prevent disease when given during incubation period.
Prophylaxis: Q fever vaccine licensed in Australia

BOTULISM

Agent: Clostridium botulinum neurotoxin (100,000 times more toxic than sarin). Could be used to sabotage food and water supplies.
Exposure: Oral or respiratory. Aerosol attack most likely.
Presentation: Incubation 1-5 days. Blocks cholinergic synapses.

Symptoms and signs: Early bulbar symptoms, weakness, paralysis, respiratory failure. Patients are usually alert, afebrile and have dry mouth.
Diagnosis: Clinical. Aerosolized toxin usually not detectable.
Isolation: Standard
Treatment: Supportive. Ventilatory support. Botulinum antitoxin more effective if given early. Trivalent/heptavalent antitoxins available through CDC or US Army.
Prophylaxis: Vaccine against inhaled botulism toxin subtypes may become available.

SEB TOXIN

Agent: Staphylococcal enterotoxin B a common cause food poisoning. Toxin is heat stable and stable in aerosols.
Exposure: Oral or respiratory. With inhalation event large % of exposed would get sick. Also, causes symptoms at low levels of exposure, incapacitating those miles from release point.
Presentation: Incubation 1-6 hours.
Symptoms and signs: Fever (lasts up to 5 days), headache, chills, myalgias, cough, nausea, vomiting, diarrhea. Rarely fatal. Patients often don't return to normal for 2 weeks.
Diagnosis: Clinical and epidemiological. Toxin usually not detectable. ELISA of nasal swabs or urine possibly. Clinically SEB will stabilize, other bioterror agents progress.
Isolation: Standard
Treatment: Supportive. Most recover in 1 week
Prophylaxis: Vaccine in development

CONCLUSION

If you have a known bioterror event, there are 10 critical steps to follow.

1. Maintain a high index of suspicion.
2. Protect yourself and your patients.
3. Adequately assess patients.
4. Decontaminate as appropriate.
5. Establish a diagnosis.
6. Provide prompt treatment.
7. Provide good infection control.
8. Alert proper authorities.
9. Assist in epidemiologic investigations.
10. Know and spread information.

Always maintain a high index of suspicion for bioterrorism. Multiple patients presenting with hemoptysis may have plague; with flaccid paralysis – botulism; with purpura – VHF; with widened mediastinum – anthrax; with centripetal rash – smallpox. And always think clinically. If patients have pulmonary symptoms, think tularemia, plague, SEB; neuromuscular symptoms – botulinum, encephalitides; bleeding – VHF, plague (late); rash – VHF, plague, smallpox; flu-like symptoms – smallpox, anthrax, tularemia, plague, SEB. Remember that doxycycline can be used to treat virtually all likely intentionally disseminated bacterial pathogens.

In the emergency department there are special problems which must be carefully addressed. Decontamination of all potentially exposed patients must be performed. Removal of clothing with soap and water cleansing is usually enough. Dilute bleach solution may be used for clothes. The risk of secondary transmission must be reduced, especially with suspected smallpox, plague or VHF. All patients with respiratory illness should be considered infectious until the organism is identified. Standard universal precautions are appropriate for most bioterror agents. Consider prophylaxis for health care workers against plague, anthrax, Q fever, smallpox. In addition, emergency departments must have a plan to appropriately allocate resources, including ventilators, protective equipment, isolations rooms, medications and vaccines.

Emergency departments should prepare for biological attacks by ensuring that medical staff are familiar with likely agents and symptoms. Bioterrorism should be incorporated into hospital disaster planning. Plans should be prepared for decontamination of patients and use of protective gear. Guidelines should be established for notification of public health agencies and law enforcement. Preparations should made for security and crowd control, and for briefing the media. Physicians, nurses and other staff should know where to obtain antibiotics and vaccines.

Research on bioterrorism is active and may enhance the ability of a population to protect itself from biological attack. Detection systems are in development that can sample and concentrate air to detect biological agents. Advanced diagnostics may yield newer and faster ways to confirm the diagnosis of bioterror agents like anthrax. New vaccines to protect against smallpox, ebola, botulism, tularemia, anthrax, Q fever, and plague are under development. New drug therapies, especially antivirals may expand treatment options for hemorrhagic fevers and the viral encephalitides. Improved skin and mucosal barriers may enhance protection of the health care worker. In addition, research can assess and improve the capacity of a health care system to respond to a bioterror event.

REFERENCES

1. *CDC. Update*: Investigation of Bioterrorism Related Anthrax and Interim Guidelines for Exposure Management and Antimicrobial Therapy,
2. October, 2001. *MMWR Weekly Report*. 2001;50(42):909-919.
3. Inhalational Anthrax among Postal Workers in Washington, D.C., and New Jersey. *The New York City Department of Health. Alert #5.* October 25,2001.
4. Torok TJ, Tauxe RV, Wise RP, et al. A Large Community Outbreak of Salmonellosis Caused by Intentional Restaurant Salad Bars. *JAMA*.1997;278(5):389-395.
5. Meselson M, Guillemin J, Hanna P. Anthrax. *N Engl J Med*.1999;341:815-26.
6. Bush LM, Abrams BH, Beall A, Johnson CC. Index Case of Fatal Inhalational Anthrax Due to Bioterrorism in the United States. *N Engl J Med* 2001;345(22):1607-1610.
7. Jernigan JA, Stephens DS, Ashford DA, et al. Bioterrorism Related Inhalational Anthrax: The First 10 Cases Reported in the United States. *Emerging Infectious Diseases*. 2001;7(6):933-944.
8. CDC. Notice to Readers: Considerations for Distinguishing Influenza-Like Illness from Inhalational Anthrax. *MMWR*. 2001;50(44):984-986
9. Inglesby TV, Henderson DA, Bartlett JG et al. Anthrax as a Biological Weapon. *JAMA*

    1999;281(18):1735-1745.
10. Franz DR, Jahrling PB, Friedlander AM, Hoover DL, et.al. Clinical Recognition and Management of
    Patients Exposed to Biological Warfare Agents. *JAMA*. 1997;278:399-411.
11. Christopher GW, Cieslak TJ, Pavlin JA, Eitzen EM. Biological Warfare, A Historical Perspective.
    JAMA. 1997;278:412-417.
12. Macintyre AG, Christopher GW, Eitzen EM, Gum R, et.al. Weapons of Mass Destruction Events
    With Contaminated Casualties: Effective Planning for Health Care Facilities. *JAMA*. 2000;283:242-249.

FOOD POISONING

John D. Cahill, M.D. & Scott Durgin, M.D.*

INTRODUCTION

Acute gastrointestinal illness, ranging from mild discomfort to life threatening sickness, is the second most common disorder worldwide. Although the actual number of food borne illness is unknown, hundreds of illnesses are capable of transmission through food. There are a medley of etiologic agents including bacteria, viruses, and toxins. The diagnosis of all food borne illness is based upon early recognition of a characteristic clinical presentation in association with a certain time frame and potentially contaminated food. This chapter will review the agents that the emergency medicine physician should be aware of.

STAPHYLOCOCCAL FOOD POISONING

Staphylococcus aureus is one of the common pathogens responsible for food borne illness worldwide. These gram-positive cocci manufacture several distinct, heat stable enterotoxins, any of which can be accountable for an outbreak. The toxins are formed prior to ingestion and therefore cause symptoms rapidly. *S. aureus* food poisoning occurs after food is left inadequately stored at temperatures fostering bacterial growth. The epidemiology of outbreaks frequently reveals a food handler who has contaminated the cuisine in question. Hence, it is an essential preventative measure to ensure hygienic food preparation as well as appropriate storage. Implicated foods include custards, baked goods (particularly deserts with cream fillings), dairy products, casseroles, potato and egg salad, and salted foods, especially meats. Buffets with foods left inappropriately, are a common source of poisoning.

As one would suspect, the pre-formed enterotoxins generate symptoms rather quickly. The typical incubation period is between one and six hours, with a median time

---

* John D. Cahill, M.D., Assistant Professor of Community Health at Brown Medical School, Department of Emergency Medicine/Rhode Island Hospital, Department of Infectious Diseases/The Miriam Hospital, Providence, Rhode Island
Scott Durgin, M.D., Dept. of Emergency Medicine/Rhode Island Hospital, Providence, Rhode Island

to presentation of four hours. The symptoms consist of profound nausea and vomiting. Non-bloody diarrhea and fever may also be noted in some patients. The syndrome is self-limited and resolves over 12-24 hours.

The diagnosis is usually clinical, although there are assays available to detect and determine specific enterotoxins. In addition, culturing of vomit, stool, suspect food, and food handler lesions may assist in identifying the origin of an outbreak. Therapy is supportive in nature and based upon the severity of symptoms. In more severe cases, intravenous fluids and anti-emetics may be necessary.

BACILLUS CEREUS FOOD POISONING

Bacillus cereus is an aerobic, spore-forming, gram-positive rod that is ubiquitous throughout the environment and is therefore frequently a food contaminant. These bacteria construct multiple different toxins that are responsible for two distinct illness patterns. Similar to other food borne illness, *B. cereus* poisoning is often associated with inadequately prepared and stored meals, where conditions favor growth of initially small bacterial contaminants. Again hygienic food preparation and good refrigeration, before and after cooking, are important preventative measures. *Bacillus cereus* poisoning has historically been associated with fried rice, being referred to as the "Chinese fried rice syndrome". Other foods commonly implicated include vegetables and meats.

As eluded to, *B. cereus* causes two types of food borne sickness as a direct result of different toxins. A heat stable toxin produced by the bacteria before consumption causes a syndrome of harsh abdominal cramps, nausea and vomiting. The symptoms present within minutes to hours and last up to 24 hours, thus the illness may mimic that of the *S. aureus* enterotoxin. Of note, the emetic toxin has a reported association with fulminant hepatic failure. The other illness caused by *B. cereus* results from a heat labile enterotoxin formed in vivo. These symptoms develop after an incubation period of 6-16 hours and include abdominal cramping and profuse diarrhea, without vomiting. This illness is also self-limiting and corrects over 24-36 hours. It is important to note that patients suffering from the emetic illness will frequently develop diarrhea.

As is typical of food poisoning, the diagnosis is clinical. Cultures and immune assays of food, vomit, and diarrhea may assist in identification of *B. cereus*. Therapy is supportive and directed at symptomatic relief.

CLOSTRIDIUM PERFRINGENS FOOD POISONING

Clostridium perfringens is a leading culprit in food borne illness, with rare, but potentially fatal complications. *Clostridium perfringens* is a spore forming anaerobic, gram-positive rod that is found in soil throughout the world. Food borne illness results from ingesting an inoculum of bacteria that subsequently produces an enterotoxin within the gastrointestinal tract. Foods that are cooked and then inadequately stored are of particular risk, as heating favors germination of the spores. High-risk foods include red meats, poultry, gravies, soups and stews.

After a person ingests a tainted meal, the enterotoxin is formed and begins damaging epithelial cells along the gastrointestinal tract. Symptoms of severe abdominal cramping and non-bloody diarrhea begin 8-16 hours later. Vomiting and fever are rare. Fortunately the illness is self limited, and symptoms should abate over 24 hours.

Diagnosis of this illness can be challenging. Clinical suspicion is mainstay, but culturing suspected food samples as well as enterotoxin testing of food and stool are available. Therapy is supportive with a focus on fluid and electrolyte balance and observation for potential complications.

Rarely, the ingestion of *C. perfringens* (type C) in conditions conducive to its growth within the intestines can cause a necrotizing enteritis known as pig-bel. Although pig-bel can be seen anywhere, it is more common in developing countries and is best known for the outbreaks in Papua New Guinea after the traditional "pig kill".

BOTULISM

Botulism is one of the most important food borne illnesses because of its' potentially fatal consequences. Recently, botulism has received significant attention due to its potential use as a weapon of terror. Regardless of its origin, a botulism outbreak constitutes a public health emergency. Every effort must be made to expeditiously identify cases to allow effective therapy and to prevent further threat to the public. *Clostridium botulinum* are anaerobic, spore-forming, gram-positive rods that exist everywhere in topsoil. Spores are heat resistant and can survive poorly undertaken food preservation. Food borne botulism occurs when victims ingest neurotoxin created by bacteria that have germinated from spores within insufficiently processed food.   The most common source is home canned goods when substandard cooking and canning methods allow spore survival, germination, and bacterial growth in an anaerobic environment where toxin production flourishes. Smoked fish is associated with type E toxin formed by a *C. botulinum* strain common to marine sediment. Unfortunately, tainted foods may not appear, smell or taste unusual.

Botulinum toxin is one of the most potent lethal substances known to man. Different strains of *C. botulinum* generate a distinct heat labile neurotoxin.   There are eight immunologic types of toxin, but human poisoning is primarily the result of types A, B, and E.   Each toxin binds irreversibly to presynaptic nerve endings inhibiting acetylcholine release, and thus producing a similar neurological syndrome.   Once formed, the toxin is subject to destruction by boiling for ten minutes or longer. Thus, sufficient cooking can prevent this illness.

Food borne botulism may initially display gastrointestinal distress including abdominal cramping, nausea, vomiting and diarrhea; but these symptoms may be absent as well. The hallmark of botulism is symmetric descending weakness and paralysis. Early neurological symptoms often manifest with cranial nerve dysfunction, consisting of diplopia, dysarthria, and/ or dysphagia.   With the onset of neurological signs and symptoms, constipation is likely to occur. Paralysis commences with the cranial nerves and descends to affect the upper extremities, the respiratory muscles, and finally the lower extremities. Signs and symptoms usually begin within 12-36 hours after exposure and may last for weeks to months. In contrast to childhood and adult botulism, infantile botulism is the result of in vivo toxin production by *C. botulinum* proliferating within the intestines. Infantile botulism has classically been associated with honey.

The diagnosis of botulism must begin with strong clinical suspicion because early therapy is of proven benefit. Botulism neurotoxin from food, vomit, stool, and serum can be detected by the mouse inoculation test performed at the CDC. Stool cultures for *C. botulinum* can also confirm a case of botulism. Ancillary testing will be of benefit to exclude other entities presenting with similar signs and symptoms: Guillain-Barre, Eaton-Lambert, and myasthenia gravis. These tests may include: magnetic resonance imaging, lumbar puncture, electromyography, and an edrophonium test.

The dominant factor that has reduced botulism mortality is comprehensive supportive care, the mainstay of which is mechanical ventilation. Pharmacological therapy exists in the form of a trivalent, equine antitoxin administered intravenously. In addition, penicillin is highly effective against *C. botulinum*, but does not destroy the toxin that has already been formed. Therefore, it is of limited use. The CDC can be contacted at anytime for diagnostic assistance and to obtain the antitoxin.

NORWALK LIKE VIRUSES

Norwalk like viruses (NLV) are non-enveloped, single stranded RNA, from the caliciviridae family or viruses. These viruses are a very important cause of gastroenteritis. The exact incidence is unknown, but the CDC estimates these viruses cause sickness in the millions. The virus frequently spreads by fecal oral transmission, by way of contaminated food and water. The source of contamination may be at food preparation, via a food handler, or at the origin of the product, such as fecal contamination of water supplies. Any food could be contaminated by Norwalk like viruses, but it is more commonly found in "ready-to-eat" foods like fruits, vegetables, salads, sandwiches, and water, even ice. Shellfish are of particular risk, as they concentrate NLV through filtration of contaminated water. Multiple food borne outbreaks of NLV have been linked to oysters.

Norwalk like viruses are relatively heat stable and can frequently survive cooking of foods. In addition, there is a very small inoculum of virus required to result in illness. After eating infected food symptoms begin within 12-48 hours, and last from 12-60 hours. Acute symptoms include nausea, vomiting, diarrhea, and abdominal cramping. Further constitutional symptoms of fever, chills, myalgias, and malaise may also be reported. Treatment is supportive, with a focus fluid and electrolyte balances. There are no long-term sequelae. Electron microscopy, immunoassays, and polymerase chain reactions have provided diagnostic tools for outbreak investigators, but are not yet of use in general practice.

HEPATITIS A

Hepatitis A primarily spreads by the fecal oral route, particularly where poor hygiene and overcrowding are prominent. The virus is often transmitted through raw shellfish and other foods contaminated by an infected food handler. Public health measures to improve hygiene are a key preventative measure.

The incubation period for hepatitis A ranges from 2-6 weeks, followed by abrupt onset of fever, malaise, prostration, nausea, vomiting, and diarrhea. After these symptoms the patient will develop dark urine, pale stools, and jaundice. The majority of patients have a self-limited illness lasting six to eight weeks. Infrequently victims may develop relapsing, cholestatic, or fulminant hepatitis A, as well as extrahepatic manifestations. In rare cases, hepatitis A can be fatal, particularly in the elderly and those patients with co-morbid liver disease.

The diagnosis of acute hepatitis A is clinical with confirmation by serologic testing. Therapy is supportive, as no specific treatment exists. Because there is no known therapy, prevention is by immunization is very important. Both passive immunization with IG and active immunization with inactivated virus exist. Passive immunization given within two weeks of exposure to hepatitis A may prevent subsequent disease in the previously un-immunized patient.

MUSHROOM POISONING

Mushroom poisoning, or mycetismus, is a common entity presenting in the warmer months of the year that support mushroom growth. Of the thousands of wild mushroom species, approximately one hundred are toxic, and about ten are potentially lethal. Mushrooms are commonly divided in different groupings based upon the toxins they contain. A thorough discussion of each mushroom toxin poisoning is beyond the scope of this chapter. The majority of mushroom fatalities are caused by the cyclopeptide containing species including amanita, galerina, and leprota mushrooms. Amatoxins are the most lethal of the cyclopeptide toxins.

Amatoxin is heat stable, water insoluble, and stable to drying, therefore it is not destroyed by food preparation. Once a mushroom is ingested, the toxin is easily absorbed and inhibits RNA polymerase 2, thereby preventing construction of vital structural proteins within cells. The most severely affected areas include centrilobular hepatocytes, gastrointestinal epithelial cells, and nephrocytes. The clinical syndrome has multiple phases, beginning with an asymptomatic phase that may last from 6-24 hours after mushroom consumption. After this latent phase the patient typically develops abdominal cramping, vomiting, and profuse diarrhea. Next the victim may clinically improve, but develop laboratory evidence of organ damage, especially hepatic injury. The final phase is one of recovery or progression to hepatic failure, with or without accompanying renal failure.

The diagnosis of amatoxin poisoning must begin with high clinical suspicion and prompt therapy must not be delayed. Amatoxin can be detected in serum, urine, and gastrointestinal fluids by a radioimmune assay. There is no specific antidote for amatoxin poisoning and the mainstay will be supportive care. Therapy should begin with gastrointestinal decontamination, including early gastric lavage followed by activated charcoal. Management of amatoxin poisoning lacks well controlled trials for specific therapies, but agents that may be beneficial include high dose penicillin and silibinin. Liver transplants can be life saving in those to progress to fulminant liver failure.

FISH POISONING

Ciguatera Poisoning

First officially described by a Portuguese biologist in the eighteenth century, ciguatera poisoning has been reported in the tropics for centuries. Although vastly under reported, ciguatera is the most common food borne syndrome related to fish worldwide. The vast majority of cases originate between 35 degrees north and south of the equator, with endemic numbers from the Caribbean and South Pacific. Heightened awareness of this affliction will allow earlier diagnosis and may assist with prevention of further cases. Hundreds of fish species have been implicated, but the most common sources are large, predatory reef dwelling fish like barracuda, grouper, and red snapper.

Multiple toxins cause Ciguatera, of which ciguatoxin is the best understood. Toxins originate in single celled organisms called dinoflagellates, which live and grow on coral reefs. Ciguatoxin, from the dinoflagellate *Gambierdiscus toxicus,* progressively bioaccumulates in the flesh and viscera of fish up the food chain. It is the larger, predatory fish that pose the risk of human poisoning. Avoidance of high-risk fish is a key preventative measure. Ciguatoxin is heat stable and unaffected by food preparation. Once absorbed the toxin displays anticholinesterase activity and opens cellular sodium channels, thereby triggering membrane depolarization. Fish are unchanged by the toxins and do no appear, taste or smell out of the ordinary.

The symptom complex can vary depending on geographic locale. Usually within 1-6 hours after ingestion patients experience abdominal cramping, nausea, vomiting, and watery diarrhea. These gastrointestinal symptoms may be preceded by, but more commonly are followed by, neurological findings including paresthesias of the mouth and throat, blurred vision, sharp shooting leg pains, and classically hot/cold temperature reversal. In addition, some people note malaise, headaches, painful/loose teeth, pruritis, myalgias, arthralgias, and dysuria. More severe poisoning may develop cranial nerve palsies, cardiovascular collapse, and even frank paralysis with respiratory failure. The neurological symptoms are the hallmark of ciguatera poisoning and typically last for days to weeks, but may persist for months.

The diagnosis is by thorough history taking and clinical findings. There is no serum toxin assay, but fish can be tested. Most cases of ciguatera sickness are self- limiting, and many people do not seek care. Therapy for the acute illness is mainly supportive with early gastrointestinal decontamination, there is no antitoxin. The use of intravenous mannitol at 1 gram per kilogram remains controversial. Although widely used with anecdotal success, a recent controlled trial failed to support any benefit in ciguatera poisoning. In severe cases, patients will require aggressive cardiovascular and respiratory resuscitation and continued support.

Persistent neurological symptoms can be a therapeutic challenge. Unfortunately there is no reliable method to predict those who will suffer prolonged symptoms, which may come to include chronic fatigue and depression. The most widely accepted therapy are tricyclic antidepressants, particularly amitryptyline. Patients should avoid alcohol, caffeine, nuts and fish for a period of six months as the substances can trigger a recurrence.

Scombroid Poisoning

Scombroid fish poisoning is one of the most common fish related illness throughout the world and was the top cause of seafood poisoning in the U.S. during the nineteen eighties. Scombroid is often unrecognized and misdiagnosed as an allergic reaction. The syndrome presents after eating dark fish meat, often from the *scombroidae* and *scomberesocidae* fish families. Poisonings have commonly been associated with tuna, bluefish, swordfish, and mahi-mahi, but has also been reported with sardines, salmon, trout, and anchovies.

Unlike other seafood illnesses, scombroid occurs from bacterial overgrowth in improperly stored fish. This mishap can frequently transpire at sea or anytime storage temperatures rise above twenty degrees Celsius for a few hours or more. At these temperatures normally small numbers of a variety of bacteria multiply. These bacteria decarboxylate histidine, which naturally resides in some fish flesh, producing histamine. After being produced histamine is not affected by cooking or freezing. Although the fish appear and smell normal, victims frequently report a peppery, salty, or bubbly taste.

The signs and symptoms of scombroid typically commence within minutes to one hour of exposure. Indeed, scombroid sickness strongly resembles an IgE mediated allergic attack. The patient begins with a warm flushing sensation and a sharply demarcated, erythematous rash develops about the face and upper torso. The rash has been described to have a burning feeling, rather than being itchy. Additional symptoms include abdominal cramps, nausea, vomiting, diarrhea, tachycardia, and occasionally bronchospasm. Symptoms left untreated resolve over 12 hours.

The diagnosis is clinical, although fish can be tested for histamine levels. Levels above 50 milligrams per 100grams of fish are likely to be toxic. Symptoms are rapidly alleviated with H1 and H2 antihistamine therapy.

Puffer Fish Poisoning

Each year, despite safeguards, puffer fish and its' associated tetrodotoxin are responsible for numerous deaths. This poisoning is most commonly witnessed in Japan and other areas where puffer fish (fugu) is considered a delicacy. The toxin responsible for this illness is tetrodotoxin, which is concentrated in the skin, viscera, and gonads of fish from the order *tetodontiformes*. Tetrodotoxin has been found in puffer fish, ocean sunfish, box fish, porcupine fish, and even some octopus, frogs, and salamanders.

Tetrodotoxin is one the most lethal natural toxins. The toxin is heat stable and unaffected by food preparation. Once consumed, tetrodotoxin inhibits nerve conduction in motor, sensory, and autonomic systems by binding sodium channels and thus preventing sodium influx. Symptoms present rapidly after ingestion and are dose dependent. Death has been reported within seventeen minutes of eating puffer fish. Early symptoms include paresthesias of the mouth and throat, followed by the extremities. Progression of the illness leads to dysarthria, dysphagia, nausea, vomiting, and weakness. Finally, in severe cases patients develop paralysis, respiratory failure, and cardiovascular collapse.

There is no definitive cure for tetrodotoxin poisoning.   Supportive therapy with early   mechanical   ventilation,   cardiovascular   resuscitation   and   gastrointestinal decontamination are mainstays. A wide range of therapies have been entertained with varying degrees of success.   Early gastric lavage with 2% sodium bicarbonate may be beneficial as the toxin is less stable in alkaline environments. Charcoal does bind the toxin and should be administered after emesis and/or lavage.   At this time other interventions are of unproven benefit.

SHELLFISH POISONING

Amnesic Shellfish Poisoning

There are numerous human illnesses that stem from pathogens and toxins concentrated in mollusks. Shellfish strain large volumes of water to nourish themselves on small organisms, which may in turn harbor bacteria, viruses, or toxins. Amnesic shellfish poisoning is caused by domoic acid that is produced by algae and subsequently concentrated in mussels and other shellfish.   This entity was first recognized in the late nineteen eighties associated with cultivated mussels off Prince Edward Island, Canada.

Domoic acid is a heat stable neuroexcitatory amino acid, which in animals has been shown to stimulate hippocampal receptors. As domoic acid is concentrated in mussel flesh there is no change in the shellfish odor, taste, or appearance.   Ingestion of contaminated shellfish produces a syndrome commencing with nausea, vomiting, diarrhea, and abdominal cramping within 24 hours. Gastrointestinal distress is followed by neurologic symptoms of confusion, disorientation, anterograde memory loss, ophthalmoplegia and in severe poisoning seizures, coma and death.   Gastrointestinal symptoms resolve over 24-48 hours, but neurological sequelae of memory loss, and motor neuropathy persist.

Diagnosis of this disease is clinical. Shellfish can be tested for domoic acid by mouse bioassays and high performance liquid chromatography.   The U.S. FDA works with multiple local officials to monitor shellfish and prevent marketing of contaminated products.   There is no specific antidote for domoic acid poisoning.   Therapy is supportive with gastrointestinal decontamination.

Paralytic Shellfish Poisoning (PSP)

Paralytic shellfish poisoning is the result of neurotoxins produced in the dinoflagellate *Protogonyaulax* and subsequently concentrated in shellfish such as mussels, clams, oysters, crabs and scallops. Poisoning related to dinoflagellates is often associated with a "red tide", a discoloration of seawater caused by high levels of these unicellular sea algae. Paralytic shellfish poisoning is primarily found in temperate climates during the warmer months of the year.

The principal toxin responsible for this shellfish illness is a heat stable molecule called saxitoxin. Saxitoxin is a compound similar to tetrodooxin and works by inhibiting sodium channels on excitatory membranes, thereby preventing nerve and muscle action potential propagation. The toxin is unaffected by cooking, freezing or other food preparation and does not alter shellfish smell, taste, or appearance.

The symptom complex of PSP is dominated by rapid onset (minutes) of neurologic complaints frequently beginning with perioral paresthesia, and then progressing to ataxia, muscle weakness, paralysis and respiratory failure. Gastrointestinal symptoms are less common. With appropriate care, symptoms usually resolve over the course of 7-10 days.

Public officials routinely monitor shellfish beds with a mouse bioassay to prevent public exposure. When cases do surface, the therapy is tailored to symptomatic control and gastrointestinal clearance.

Neurotoxic Shellfish Poisoning

Neurotoxic shellfish poisoning is caused by multiple toxins manufactured in the dinoflagellate *Ptychodiscus brevis*. This dinoflagellate is also associated with "red tides" occurring primarily in the southeastern U.S., Caribbean, and Gulf of Mexico. The shellfish most commonly implicated are clams and oysters.

Ptychodiscus brevis produce both neurotoxins and hemolytic toxins called brevetoxins. The principal activities of the brevetoxins are enhancement of sodium channel permeability, and inhibition of phagocyte protienases. Brevetoxins can cause two clinical syndromes, one after consuming contaminated shellfish and the other after inhaling aerosolized sea spray during an algal bloom.

The first illness occurs within minutes to hours of ingesting contaminated shellfish. Symptoms of abdominal pain, nausea, diarrhea and circumoral paresthesia begin quickly. Paresthesias may progress to the throat, torso and extremities with dizziness and ataxia as well. Overall the syndrome is much less severe than PSP and symptoms resolve over 24-48 hours.

A second syndrome that disserves mention presents when these same toxins are inhaled, typically during an algal bloom. The illness causes nasal and respiratory irritation with coughing, sneezing, rhinorrhea, lacrimation, shortness of breath and bronchospasm. These symptoms often dissipate upon leaving the water area. However, patients with underlying lung disease are predisposed and may require further therapy.

Therapeutic measures are again supportive as the sickness is self-limited and usually resolves within a few days.   Gastrointestinal decontamination may be of benefit for ingested toxin and bronchodilators for respiratory distress.

SEAFOOD ALLERGIES

Hypersensitivity to seafood is one of the most common food allergies. The spectrum of disease ranges from mild to life threatening. Shellfish, along with peanuts, are the most common causes of food-based anaphylaxis. Allergic reactions to seafood are IgE mediated, and like other allergic reactions manifest with pruritis and urticaria. In severe cases, the allergic reaction can rapidly progress to angioedema, vascular collapse, and/or respiratory distress due to airway edema as well as potential bronchial and laryngeal spasm.

Management is tailored to the severity of the allergic reaction. In milder cases antihistamines and glucocorticoids will alleviate symptoms and prevent disease progression. In severe presentations epinephrine is the mainstay of therapy, with aggressive airway management.

REFERENCES

1. Blakesley ML: Scombroid poisoning: prompt resolution of symptoms with cimetidine. *Annals of Emergency Medicine* 1983; 12:104-106.
2. Borriello SP: Clostridial disease of the gut. *Clinical Infectious Disease* 1995; 20(Suppl 2): 242-250.
3. Dickinson G: Scombroid fish poisoning syndrome. *Annals of Emergency Medicine* Sept 1982; 487-488
4. Holmes RJ, et al: Emetic food poisoning caused by *Bacillus cereus*. *Archives of Medicine* 1981; 141:766 -767.
5. Jong EC: Food, Fish, and Shellfish Poisoning. *Travel Medicine Advisor* 17.1-17.7
6. Kemmer NM, Miskovsky EP: Infections of the liver. Infectious Disease Clinics of North America 2000; 14(3):
7. Lange RW: Puffer fish poisoning. *American Family Physician* Oct 1990;1029-1033.
8. Lange RW: Ciguatera fish poisoning. *American Family Physician* Sept 1994; 579-584.
9. Mahler H, et al: Fulminant liver failure in association with the emetic toxin of *Bacillus cereus*. *NEJM* 1997;336(16): 11421148.
10. Mcpartland JM, Vilgays RJ, Cubeta MA: Mushroom poisoning. *American family Physician* 1997; 55(5): 1797-1809
11. Pearn J: Neurology of ciguatera. *Journal of Neurology, Neurosurgery, and Psychiatry* 2001; 70(1): 4-8.
12. Perl TM, et al: An outbreak of toic enchepalopathy caused by eating mussels contaminated with domoic acid. *NEJM* 1990; 322(25): 1775-1780.
13. Sakamoto Y, Lockey RF, Krzanowski JJ: Shellfish and fish poisoning related to the toxic dinoflagellates. *Southern Medical Journal* 1987; 80(7): 866-872.
14. Sanchez-Guerrero IM, Vidal JB, Escudero AI: Scombroid fish poisoning: A potentially life-threatening allergic like reaction. *Journal of Allergy and Clinical Immunology* 1997;433-434
15. Shapiro RL, Hatheway C, Swerdlow D: Botulism in the United States: A clinical and epidemiologic review. *Annals of Internal Medicine* 1998; 129(3): 221-228.
16. Sims JK, Ostman DC: Pufferfish Poisoning: Emergency Diagnosis and Management of mild human tetrodotoxication. *Annals of Emergency Medicine* Sept 1986; 1094-1098.
17. Teitelbaum JS, et al: Neurologic sequelae of domoic acid intoxication due to the ingestion of contaminated mussels. *NEJM* 1990; 322(25): 1781-1787.
18. Tranter HS: Foodborne staphyloccocal illness. *The Lancet* 1990; 336:1044-1046.

EVALAUTION OF THE FEBRILE TRAVELER

John D. Cahill, M.D.[*]

In the past, diseases of the tropics were considered to be exotic and not something that a physician needed to have knowledge of. However, air travel currently allows one to travel across the globe rapidly. One can be in a malaria endemic region of Africa one day, and the next day febrile in a physician's office or presenting to an Emergency Department. Each year, over 50 million people travel from the industrialized world to the developing world. It is estimated that for every 100,000 travelers who go to the developing world for one month: 50,000 will develop a health problem, 8000 will be sick enough to seek medical attention, 5000, will be confined to bed, 300 will require hospitalization, and one will die. The common presenting complaints in returned travelers are: 65% diarrhea, 24% fever, 10% skin conditions, and 1% sexually transmitted diseases[†]. This chapter will go over the evaluation of a febrile returned traveler.

HISTORY

A very thorough history is essential in the evaluation of these patients. Besides obtaining the general medical history, there are certain questions that should be asked:

- Where is the patient returning from?
- What was the season?
- How long was the trip?
- Were any other countries visited?
- What was the purpose and nature of the trip?
- What were the sleeping and living accommodations?
- Did the accommodations have air conditioning, screens, or was a mosquito net used?
- Any side trips or activities done?
- Dietary history?

[*] John D. Cahill, M.D., Assistant Professor of Community Health at Brown Medical School, Department of Emergency Medicine/Rhode Island Hospital, Department of Infectious Diseases/The Miriam Hospital, Providence, Rhode Island

- Contact with animals?
- Insect bites?
- Swimming in freshwater?
- Sexual history?
- Any medical or dental interventions?
- Before traveling were appropriate immunizations given?
- Was malaria chemoprophylaxis given and was it taken correctly?

A careful history of the fever presentation should be obtained. The time of onset can be a powerful tool in refining and limiting the differential diagnosis (table 1). Every pathogen can be characterized by a typical incubation period, the interval between exposure, and the development of clinical signs and symptoms of infection. Incubation periods can range from minutes to decades. The pattern of fever should also be inquired about. Is the fever constant, cyclical, or relapsing? Are there any associated symptoms

Table 1: Onset of Illness

Up to a week	Short Course	Intermediate:1 month	Long Course
Malaria	Malaria	Amoebiasis	Amoebiasis
Arboviruses	Meningococcus	Clonorchiais	Brucellosis
Anthrax	Plague	CMV	Hepatitis B & C
Dengue fever	Relapsing fever	Fascioliasis	Histoplasmosis
Japanese Encephalitis	Rickettsial	Hepatitis A, C, E	HIV
Legionnaire's	Typhoid	HIV	Leishmaniasis
Leptospirosis	Yellow Fever	Malaria	Malaria
		Rabies	Rabies
		Schistosomiasis	TB
		Trypanosomiasis	

with the fever? Three questions can help to focus thinking on an individual patient with a fever:

1. What is possible based on time and place of exposure?
2. What is likely based on epidemiological data, activities, host factors, and clinical and laboratory data?
3. What is treatable or transmissible or both?

The major causes of fever in returning travelers are shown in Table Two. After a history is obtained, a careful physical exam should be performed. Significant findings can help limit the differential diagnosis and therefore causes of fever will be discussed based upon clinical presentation. An organ system approach will be used to help in the evaluation. However, malaria will be considered separately due to the importance of the disease.

Table 2: Causes of Fever in the Returned Traveler

Cause	Percent
Malaria	32
Respiratory infections	11
Hepatitis	6
Diarrhea	4.5
UTI	4
Typhoid	2
Dengue	2
Unknown	25

MALARIA

Malaria must be considered in any febrile traveler returning from an endemic region. Over forty-one percent of the world's population lives in areas where malaria is transmitted (e.g. parts of Africa, Asia, Oceania, Central America, and South America). Approximately 300-500 million clinical infections occur annually, resulting in 1.5 to 2.7 million deaths. Malaria is most commonly transmitted during the bite of a female Anopheles mosquito. Humans can be infected with one of four species of *Plasmodium* (*falciparum, vivax, ovale, and malariae).*

Other means of transmission have been reported and they include: blood transfusions, intravenous drug abuse using contaminated syringes, perinatal transmission, organ transplantation, and so-called "airport malaria". There have been several reports of persons acquiring malaria who have never been in an endemic area, but live near or work in an international airport. In a recent study done looking at malaria in Rhode Island, 82% of the patients were diagnosed with *Plasmodium falciparum*. This is an important observation, since *Plasmodium falciparum* is the species responsible for most deaths and severe cases. *Plasmodium vivax* and *ovale* are unique in that they have a hypnozoite form that which allows them to remain dormant in the body for possibly months to years.

Malaria usually has an incubation period of about a week, however physicians must remember that patients can present several years later with acute illness. The patient with malaria will always have a fever, other symptoms may include: headache, cough, and gastrointestinal symptoms. Complicated malaria due to *P. falciparum* may cause: cerebral malaria, anemia, high output congestive heart failure, pulmonary edema, acute renal failure, metabolic acidosis, DIC, and hypoglycemia. The diagnosis of malaria is simply made by performing a blood film; however absence of visualization of the parasite does not exclude malaria. Oral treatment options include: Quinine and Doxycycline, Proguanil/Ataquavone, or Mefloquine. Patients who cannot tolerate oral medication or show evidence of complicated malaria should be started on intravenous Quinine or Quinidine.

Although chemoprophylaxis with antimalarials are effective, they do not guarantee protection. Current options for prophylaxis: Chloroquine (in sensitive areas), Mefloquine, Proguanil/Ataquavone, and Doxycycline.

MALAISE

The differential diagnosis of a patient complaining with malaise is tremendous. However, several diseases are well known to present with generalized malaise. Most patients with malaria present with generalized malaise that is typically worse during the febrile periods. Dengue fever has been described as aching in the bones, back, and joints. Yellow fever and the hemorrhagic fevers classically cause a "flu-like" malaise. Viral hepatitis and tuberculosis are other causes

LYMPHADENOPATHY

Dengue fever, Yellow fever, and other arboviruses can cause generalized lymphadenopathy. African Trypanosomiasis classically involves the posterior cervical lymph nodes and is known as Winterbottom's sign. Visceral Leishmaniasis may cause lymphadenopathy, especially in patients from the Sudan. Tuberculosis can cause generalized lymphadenopathy, but has a predilection for the cervical lymph nodes and is known as scrofula. Plague caused from Yersinia pestis usually forms buboes in the femoral and inguinal lymph nodes. Infection with the filarial worm Wuchereria bancrofti or Brugia malayi often involve the groin or axillary nodes. It should be noted that filariais is not a disease of travelers, but one of individuals who live in an endemic region. It should be remembered that primary HIV infection can present with lymphadenopathy.

JAUNDICE

Any common cause of viral hepatitis should be considered: EBV, Hepatitis A, B, C, D, or E, and CMV. Malaria causes jaundice secondary to massive hemolysis. Significant cases of *Leptospira icterohemorrhagia* can cause jaundice. Although Yellow Fever is extremely rare in the USA, in it's second phase it causes a significant hepatitis. Yellow Fever can be differentiated from the other viral causes of hepatitis by the AST transaminase being higher than ALT. The opposite holds true for other viral causes of hepatitis. It is important to always ask about any medications, alcohol, or toxins that could cause hepatitis.

HEPATOMEGALY

- Viral Hepatitis
- Malaria
- Visceral Leishmaniasis
- Amoebiasis
- Hydatid Cyst

SPLENOMEGALY

- Malaria
- Visceral Leishmaniasis
- Typhoid Fever
- Brucellosis
- Bartonellosis
- Acute Chagas Disease
- African Trypanosomiasis
- Viral Infections
- Neoplastic process

DIARRHEA

The evaluation of diarrhea in the returned traveler should be approached in a systematic fashion. This discussion will be limited to the febrile patient with diarrhea. Diarrhea can be divided by history and exam into bloody and non-bloody. The most common causes of non-bloody diarrhea would be: salmonella enteritis, malaria (especially in children), mild shigellosis, and campylobacter. For bloody diarrhea: shigella, campylobacter enterocolitis, typhoid, and verotoxin producing strains of *E. coli.*

NEUROLOGICAL

Meningitis is still a common cause of infection worldwide. Besides the common bacterial causes, fungal, viral, and tuberculosis must be considered in these patients. Cerebral malaria can present as headache, seizure, lethargy, and coma. Typhoid fever can present with a change in mental status or what has been described as a "typhoid state". CNS symptoms are not common in acute African Trypanosomiasis, although they can occur.

DERMATOLOGICAL

Many tropical diseases can present with dermatological findings. Patients infected with typhoid fever may present with rose spots, pink macules on the trunk which are only usually noted in fair- skinned individuals. Rickettsial infections present with a maculopapular rash over the trunk which spreads to the extremities. The rash in dengue fever presents in a similar fashion as the rickettsial infections. In Chagas' disease there may be initial orbital edema (Romana's sign) or an area of cutaneous edema may develop known as a chagoma. In Leptospirosis a transient urticarial, macular, maculopapular, erythematous, or purpuric rash may develop. Outside of the USA, syphilis is still quite common and should be considered in one's differential of a rash. Helminths can cause a variety of skin manifestations, which are beyond the scope of this paper.

INITIAL EVALUATION

After a careful history and physical, laboratory results can help limit the differential diagnosis. At minimum all febrile sick travelers should have a CBC with differential, LFT's, Blood Cultures, Urinalysis, Blood film, and have extra tubes drawn for serology. Patients with respiratory symptoms should have a CXR and a sputum sample sent for gram stain and AFB. Patients with diarrhea should have stool examined for fecal leukocytes, ova and parasites, and a stool culture sent. Further testing can be done as deemed appropriate.

Eosinophilia can be caused from infectious sources, allergic disease states, and hematological and neoplastic processes. The physician should always think of non-infectious causes before engaging in the million dollar work up. Helminths are the most common infectious cause of eosinophilia. Protozoan infections such as malaria do not typically cause eosinophilia. One must remember that multiple infections may be present and that the absence of eosinophilia does not exclude parasitic infection.

In conclusion, there are several key points to remember in the evaluation of these patients:

1. Fever after travel may be unrelated to exposures during travel.
2. Always think of malaria.
3. Exposure to many widely distributed infections is more common during travel than during life at home.
4. Re-examine the febrile patient if the initial evaluation does not suggest a specific diagnosis.
5. Keep in mind the public health implications.

REFERENCES

1. International Society of Travel Medicine Introduction to Travel Medicine:Slide Lecture Kit, slide 4, 1998 Stone Mountain
2. Caumes E. *Health and Travel*:1999 Edition, p118-119, Pasteur Merieux MSD
3. Guerrant RL, Walker DH, Weller PF. Tropical Infectious Diseases: Principles, Pathogens, & Practice. p1383 1st ed. 1999, Churchill Livingstone, Philadelphia
4. Danis M, Gentilini M. Malaria, a worldwide scourge. *Rev Prat* 1998 Feb 1:48(3):254-7.
5. Van den Ende J, Lynen L, Elsen P, Colebunders R, Demey H, Depraetere K, De Schrijver K, Peetermans WE, Pereira de Almeida P, Vogelaers D. A cluster of airport malaria in Belgium in 1995. *Acta Clin Belg* 1998 Aug;53(4):259-63.
6. Cahill JD, Mileno M, et al. Malaria in Rhode Island: Observations From 1990-1998, Journal of Travel Medicine, *Journal of Travel Medicine* 2001;8:100-102
7. Guerrant RL, Walker DH, Weller PF. Tropical Infectious Diseases: Principles, Pathogens, & Practice. p1401, 1st ed. 1999, Churchill Livingstone, Philadelphia

APPROACH TO THE POISONED PATIENT

John D. Cahill, M.D.[*]

Treating ingestions whether purposeful or not, is a skill every emergency medicine physician must have. One must always think of possible toxicological causes for the presentation of a patient with unexplained signs or symptoms. The physician who misses a significant acetaminophen overdose on first presentation, has little ground to stand on when the patient returns in liver failure. This chapter will go over the approach to the poisoned patient and then present several cases, stressing critical points.

As one was told repeatedly in medical school, the history is 85% of the key to making a diagnosis. This holds especially true when evaluating a toxicological exposure. If the patient is awake and cooperative, the history may be obtained from them. Otherwise one needs to rely on family, friends, co-workers, rescue personnel, or pharmacies to try to obtain the history. Useful information to know: time of ingestion, quantity, dose, multiple substances taken, what were the circumstances (gardening, home, at work) where the patient was found, and any events leading to the ingestion? When there is a question of potential suicide attempt, the physician needs to be very aware of the patient possibly minimizing the ingestion or the event. More than once, suicidal patients have down played life threatening ingestions as "I just took a couple of pills".

When a patient arrives to the emergency department with a poisoning, one should always remember to protect themselves, department staff, and the other patients. Does the patient need to be decontaminated? If so, this should be done away from the rest of the department and appropriate gear should be used. If the patient is agitated or possibly violent, appropriate restraints should be used (verbal, chemical, or physical). With all patients in the emergency department, the "ABC's" are first priority. During the physical exam any evidence of specific toxidromes should be looked for. One should remember that the sense of smell may be of particular use. Certain substances give off a particular odor: cyanide- almonds, arsenic - garlic, chloral hydrate - pears, and nitrobenzene- shoe polish, to mention a few.

[*] John D. Cahill, M.D., Assistant Professor of Community Health at Brown Medical School, Department of Emergency Medicine/Rhode Island Hospital, Department of Infectious Diseases/The Miriam Hospital, Providence, Rhode Island

Except for immediate life threatening oral ingestions that present within one hour, gastric lavage is not indicated. Activated charcoal is felt to be of some benefit in oral ingestions. The usual dose is 50 grams of activated charcoal; it works by adsorbing most drugs & chemicals. A cathartic may enhance transit time of charcoal: sorbitol or magnesium citrate. Multidose charcoal may be useful in enhancing elimination of drugs already absorbed. It should be remembered that activated charcoal is ineffective against: Ions (mineral acids & alkalis, lithium, borates, bromides), Hydrocarbons, Metals, and Ethanol. In these circumstances, one may consider whole bowel irrigation with polyethylene glycol.

Whenever there is a concern for a significant ingestion or exposure, IV access should be established. Besides supportive treatment, other modalities of treatment for poisoning may include: intubation, specific antidote use (table 1), chelation therapy, alkalization of urine, hemodialysis, and hemoperfusion.

Table 1: Specific Antidotes

Agent	Antidote
Opiates	Naloxone
Benzodiazepines	Flumazenil
Tricyclic Antidepressants	$NaHCO_3$
Anticholinergic	Physostigmine
Cholinergic	Atropine/Pralidoxime
Calcium Channel Blockers	Calcium
Beta Blockers	Glucagon
Digoxin	Digoxin specific FAB fragments
Acetaminophen	N-acetylcysteine
Methanol	Ethanol/Fomepizole, Folate or Leucovorin
Ethylene Glycol	Ethanol/Fomepizole, Thiamine & Pyridoxine
Isoniazid	Pyridoxine
Cyanide	Amyl nitrite, Sodium nitrite &Sodium thiosulfate
Iron	Deferoxamine
Lead	EDTA, DSMA, Dimercaprol (BAL), D-Penicillamine
Arsenic	Dimercaprol (BAL), D-Penicillamine
Mercury	Dimercaprol (BAL), D-Penicillamine
Snake Venom	Monovalent or Polyvalent Antivenom

Depending on the presentation of the patient, certain laboratory studies may be warranted. In the case of the unknown ingestion or suicide attempt, an aspirin and acetaminophen level should always be drawn. Electrolytes can be useful to look for the presence of an anion gap (table 2), renal function, and glucose. Liver function tests may of use to demonstrate baseline function or hepatic injury. In more severe ingestions, an arterial blood gas may be helpful. An electrocardiogram should be obtained when there is evidence or concern about possible ingestion of: tricyclic antidepressant, cardiac medication overdoses (beta-blockers, digoxin, calcium channel blockers), quinine, cocaine/amphetamine use, persistent tachycardia/bradycardia, and a significant change in mental status. A urinalysis can aid in the diagnosis of ethylene glycol ingestion when the presence of calcium oxalate crystals is noted. A pregnancy test should be done on all females of child bearing age. A serum osmolality may help discern the evidence of a volatile alcohol ingestion. Other specific levels and toxicological screens can be sent as warranted. A chest x-ray may help demonstrate noncardiogenic pulmonary edema in salicylate or opiate toxicity. A KUB can help visualize heavy metals, chloral hydrate, phenothiazines, and smuggled packets.

Table 2: Causes of an Increased Anion Gap

M	Methanol
U	Uremia
D	Diabetic Ketoacidosis
P	Paraldehyde
I	Isoniazid & Iron
L	Lactic Acidosis
E	Ethylene Glycol
S	Salicylates

Disposition on these patients can often become an issue and although not absolute, one can usually discharge home the following patients after a 4-6 hour observation:

- no admission of feeling suicidal
- no overt signs of toxicity after decontamination and administration of activated charcoal
- the toxic agent ingested is not a sustained-release product
- methanol: no evidence of acidosis, blood levels below 10 mg/dL,
- in tricyclic antidepressant poisoning with no tachycardia, QRS widening, anticholinergic symptoms or drowsiness

Criteria to admit patients includes the following, but is not limited to:

- all suicide attempts (obtain psychiatric consultation)
- life-threatening signs and symptoms
- manifestations of allergy or hypersensitivity
- any ingestion of unknown amounts of a potentially dangerous poison in a child
- symptomatic methemoglobinemia in children (levels over 20% in patients requiring methylene blue administration)
- symptomatic child with acute neuroleptic poisoning
- snakebites requiring antivenom

- body stuffers of cocaine until all packets are passed
- any patient requiring hyperbaric oxygen who exhibits an acidosis
- carboxyhemoglobin level greater than 20% after carbon monoxide exposure
- ingestion of acetonitrile-containing compounds
- paralytic shellfish poisoning or tetrodotoxin exposure with respiratory depression
- hydrocarbons: symptoms during first 6 hours of observation after a hydrocarbon ingestion
- iron: child requiring intravenous chelation for iron poisoning
- symptomatic patients of Isoniazid poisoning

CASE 1

A 23 year old female was brought into the ED by her family stating "what's the big deal, I took a bottle of pain killers 1 hour ago when I was mad at my boyfriend". Her vital signs and physical exam are normal. What is your approach to this patient? What tests if any would you order? All the following tests ordered were within normal limits: electrolytes, alcohol, drugs of abuse, pregnancy test negative, electrocardiogram, and a salicylate level. An acetaminophen level at 1.5 hour was 200mg/L and the 4 hour was 300mg/L. When plotted on the nomogram, this was noted to be a significant overdose requiring treatment.

In general taking more than 7.5g in an adult or 140mg/kg of acetaminophen in a 24 hour period is hepatotoxic. Acetaminophen causes hepatotoxicity by being metabolized by the P450 system to the toxic metabolite:N-acetyl-para-benzoquinoneimine (NAPQI). Four stages of Acetaminophen poisoning have been described:

(1) 0-24h nausea, vomiting
(2) 24-48h abdominal pain, increasing LFT's
(3) 72-96h LFT's peak, nausea, vomiting
(4) 4d – 14d resolution or hepatic failure.

Initial treatment is with activated charcoal which significantly decreases absorption if given within 2 hours of ingestion. There is no role for multidose activated charcoal, especially if the antidote acetylcysteine is going to be given. Acetylcysteine can be given orally or intravenously: loading dose 140mg/kg then 70mg/kg every 4 hours x 17 doses. To date, only the oral dosing has been approved by the FDA for use in the USA, however much of Europe uses the intravenous form. The intravenous form may be preferred to guarantee delivery without the risk of vomiting (especially if you have ever smelled acetylcysteine) or in people with a change in mental status. If the oral dose is given, it should be repeated if the patient vomits within one hour of the dose. The utility of acetylcysteine is controversial if given after 24 hours post ingestion.

CASE 2

A 26 year old female took a bottle of her "depression pills" & drank a fifth of whisky, initially extremely agitated, she then became comatose. Her vital signs are remarkable for a temperature of 39 Celsius, sinus tachycardia in the 120's, hypotensive with a blood pressure of 85/40, and a respiratory rate in the upper 20's. Physical exam is remarkable for dry mucous membranes, no gag reflex & flushed skin. An electrocardiogram shows sinus tachycardia with widening of the QRS. A Foley catheter was placed with a return of 30cc of urine. How would you manage this patient and what is in your differential diagnosis?

This patient is presenting with a Tricyclic antidepressant overdose. Significant Tricyclic overdoses must be managed aggressively to avoid death. One should always start with the ABC's as IV access is being established and the patient is placed on a monitor. Gastric lavage may be indicated if the patient has had a significant ingestion within one hour prior to arrival. Otherwise activated charcoal should be given. Sodium Bicarbonate should be given when any of the following are present:

- QRS >100ms
- cardiac dysrhythmias
- seizures
- hypotension.

The goal is to maintain a pH of 7.5. Seizures can be treated with benzodiazepines or phenobarbital. The mainstay of treatment for hypotension is fluids and the diligent use of vasopressors. Norepinephrine and phenylephrine are the pressors of choice due to their alpha adrenergic properties.

This patient presented with a toxidrome classic for anticholinergic poisoning. Common anticholinergic agents include: cyclic antidepressants, antihistamines, phenothiazines, scopolamine, belladonna, jimson weed, nightshade, and Amanita muscaria mushrooms. The signs and symptoms of anticholenegeric poisoning can be remembered by the saying "hot as a hare, blind as a bat, dry as a bone, red as a beet, mad as a hatter."

Since one is mentioning anticholinergic poisoning, one can include a discussion on cholinergic poisoning. Cholinergic poisoning is commonly seen with pesticides and as potential weapons of mass destruction. Cholinergic agents can broadly be divided into organophosphate inhibitors and Carbamates. Organophosphate inhibitors bind irreversibly to cholinesterase inhibitors, are longer acting, and may demonstrate CNS toxicity. Carbamates are reversible inhibitors, shorter acting, and demonstrate no CNS toxicity. Both are absorbed via the skin, conjunctiva, lungs, and from the GI tract.

The diagnosis is made by history, recognizing the toxidrome (table 3), or in the laboratory by confirmation of the presence of plasma cholinesterase/RBC acetyl cholinesterase. Treatment is by decontamination and using atropine until signs of effect are recognized. Pralidoxime may be used in the case of severe organophosphate poisoning.

Table 3: Cholinergic Presentation

D	Diarrhea
U	Urination
M	Miosis
B	Bronchospam
E	Emesis
L	Lacrimation
S	Salivation

CASE 3

A 32 year old male with a PMHX of alcohol abuse presents stating "This booze is so sweet, that a day later I cannot even see". The agent to be concerned about in this case is methanol. It is not uncommon for individuals to drink methanol if they cannot get their hands on ethanol. A brief review of the volatile alcohols will be discussed.

Methanol is sweet tasting and colorless. It can be found in a variety of products: antifreeze, windshield washer fluid, carburetor fluid, duplicator fluid, gasohol, sterno, and in multiple thinners. The metabolism of methanol is noted in figure one.

Clinically patients can present with: GI upset, headache, depressed mental status, confusion, ocular toxicity (retinal edema, hyperemia of disc, documentation of visual acuity is essential), and a metabolic acidosis: which may occur 12-24hrs later.

Figure 1: Metabolism of Methanol

Methanol
                                                              ↓ Alcohol Dehydrogenase

                                        Formaldehyde
                            ↓ Alcohol Dehydrogenase

                                        Formic Acid

                ↓ Folate

              Carbon Dioxide & Water

Ethylene Glycol is found in antifreeze and failure to recognize may result in death in 24-36 hours later. It only takes a few ml/kg to be fatal. Clinically patients may present with: CNS intoxication, drunk without the smell of ETOH, GI upset, metabolic acidosis, cardiac instability, and renal failure. The metabolism of ethylene glycol is shown in figure two.

Figure 2: Ethylene Glycol Metabolism

```
Ethylene glycol
              ↓Alcohol Dehydrogenase

Glycoaldehyde
              ↓Aldehyde Dehydrogenase

Glycolic Acid

↓
Glyoxylic Acid

        ↓ Pyridoxine     ↓      ↓           ↓Thiamine

      Glycine       Oxalate   Formic Acid  Alpha-Hydroxy-Beta-
                                            Ketoadipate (Non toxic)
```

Diagnosing methanol and ethylene glycol ingestion is done by taking a good history, looking for physical exam finding, and on a laboratory basis. An anion gap with a metabolic acidosis is almost always seen. A serum osmolal gap greater than 10mOsm is also suggestive. One can calculate the expected Osmolal gap by the formula:

2 x Na (mEq/L) + glucose (mg/dl)/18 +BUN (mg/dl)/2.8 + ethanol (mg/dl)/4.3

A volatile alcohol screen is obviously helpful, although one should not withhold treatment if clinical suspicion is high for ingestion of either. In ethylene glycol ingestion the urine can be examined to look for the presence of Calcium Oxalate crystals or fluorescence under a Wood's lamp.

Gastric lavage may be useful if ingestion has occurred within 30-60min. Activated charcoal has no role in the management of these ingestions. Sodium Bicarbonate may be used to treat the acidosis. In both cases, Ethanol or Fomepizole competitively blocks the metabolism of alcohol dehydrogenase and therefore limits the production of toxic metabolites. Hemodialysis will also aid in removing the preformed toxic metabolites. Hemodialysis is usually indicated with a level above 25mg/dl.

Isopropyl Alcohol is found in rubbing alcohol and gained recognition when one of our former presidential candidate's wives chose it as her favorite spirit. It is not as toxic as the other volatile alcohols. Isopropyl alcohol is metabolized to acetone. It can be twice as intoxicating as alcohol and is a significant gastric irritant. Metabolic acidosis is not usually seen. In most cases, treatment is supportive only, rarely hemodialysis may be required.

REFERENCES

1. Olson KR, Pentel PR, Kelley MT: Physical assessment and differential diagnosis of the poisoned patient, *Med Toxicol* 2:52, 1987.
2. Goldfrank L: Teaching the recognition of odors, *Ann Emerg Med* 11:684, 1982.
3. *Rosen's Emergency Medicine: Concepts and Clinical Practice, 5th ed.*, Mosby, St.Louis p.2068
4. Smilkstein MJ: Acetaminophen. In Goldfrank LR et al, editors: *Goldfrank's toxicologic emergencies,* ed 6, Stamford, Conn, 1998, Appleton & Lange.
5. Ellison DW, Pentel PR: Clinical features and consequences of seizures due to cyclic antidepressant overdose, *Am J Emerg Med* 7:5, 1989.
6. Shannon M, Merola J, Lovejoy FH: Hypotension in severe tricyclic antidepressant overdose, *Am J Emerg Med* 6:439, 1988.
7. Jacobsen D, McMartin KE: Methanol and ethylene glycol poisonings: mechanism of toxicity, clinical course, diagnosis and treatment, *Med Toxicol* 1:309–334, 1986.
8. Jacobsen D, McMartin KE: Antidotes for methanol and ethylene glycol poisoning, *Clin Toxicol* 35:127–143, 1997.

PSYCHIATRIC EMERGENCIES

Walter Simmons, M.D., M.P.H.[*]

As an aid to understanding the approach and treatment of patients suffering from psychiatric illnesses in the emergency department, it is beneficial to first have an appreciation of the people who have played a key role in developing modern-day psychiatry. Dr. Benjamin Rush (1745-1813) is an example of one person that made an addition to the field of psychiatric medicine and can be considered a hero in psychiatry. Dr. Rush, an American who graduated from the University of Edinburgh, Scotland in 1766 served on the Pennsylvania Hospital medical staff from 1783 until the year of his death in 1813. In this position, he wore many hats. He was the first American professor of chemistry, a signer of the Declaration of Independence, a pioneer abolitionist, and a proponent of prison reform. Foremost he was considered by many to be the father of American psychiatry. It is believed Rush wrote the first psychiatric textbook to be printed in the U.S entitled *Observations and Inquiries upon the Diseases of the Mind*, published in 1812. Rush's book contains several astute insights regarding psychiatry, including that mental illness is a disease of the mind. The book also contains Rush's beliefs regarding the influence of buried memories, the importance of psychiatric training in general medical education, the holistic unity of body and mind, and the recognition that emotions and behavior, as well as intellect, can suffer derangement. In the words of his biographer Dr. Carl Binger, "he took on heroic stature, substituting kindness and compassion for cruelty, and replacing routine reliance on archaic procedures by careful clinical observation and study."

With an increased awareness regarding one of psychiatry's forefathers, let's move on to discuss some of the interesting epidemiology of emergency psychiatric medicine. Approximately 15% of patients seen in the emergency department (ED) present with a chief complaint that is strongly related to a psychiatric illness. It has been shown, that the presentation of patients with psychiatric complaints rise dramatically between the hours of midnight to 8 am, with as much as 50% of all patient visits to the ED having a psychiatric component. In addition, certain groups seen in an emergency setting may suffer a higher prevalence of mental illness. Of the homeless visiting the ED, 20-40% suffer from a major mental illness.

---

[*] Walter N. Simmons, M.D., M.P.H., Fellow in Emergency Medicine, Brown University/Rhode Island Hospital

With the number of patients seen with true psychiatric illness, a large problem faced by emergency physicians is distinguishing between a psychiatric illness and an illness with an organic basis. As proof of the difficulty in this effort, it has been shown that 30% of patients sent to a psychiatric hospital are found to have an organic basis for their illness.

Case studies can aid in the teaching of patient care and can be a challenge to the reader's intellect. Therefore, several cases will be presented. The reader should read each case carefully and attempt to answer the questions presented as an educational exercise. This chapter is not designed or meant to be a full review of all the psychiatric presentations to the emergency department. Instead, the chapter will focus on a few topics often encountered by a physician operating in an emergency setting. In particular, the chapter will concentrate on schizophrenia, depression, mania, and anxiety.

FIRST CASE STUDY

A 50-year-old male who is a well-known powerful political figure in the area is brought in by rescue. When found by the paramedics, the man was running naked through the streets. Upon talking to this person in the ED, you find him to be restless, confused, and to have racing thoughts. What would be a general approach to this patient?

The patient described above is loosely based upon the presentation of King George III (1760-1820) during a time of madness. King George III has created a place in history for both losing the American colonies and going mad during his reign of England. Although the patient presented may suffer solely from a psychiatric illness, we must always be reminded of the high cost of missing organic causes for psychiatric illness. In this case, the basis for the patient's mental state is caused by the hereditary disease, acute intermittent porphyria. This is a disease that also tormented Mary Queen of Scots, who passed it on to her son, King James I of England.

Acute intermittent porphyria is an autosomal dominant disorder most frequently seen in women. The disease is a diagnostic quagmire mimicking a variety of commonly occurring disorders. Porphyria most often presents with complaints of abdominal pain and motor paralysis. Psychiatric manifestations may include: hysteria, anxiety, depression, phobias, psychosis, organic disorders, agitation, delirium, and altered consciousness ranging from somnolence to coma. The disease is known to masquerade as a psychosis or personality disorder and there are documented cases of these patients being treated as schizophrenics or as a patient suffering from a histrionic personality disorder.

The diagnosis of acute intermittent porphyria can be entertained in the following situations: unexplained leukocytosis, unexplained neuropathy, etiologically obscure neurosis or psychosis, 'idiopathic' seizure disorder, unexplained abdominal pain, conversion hysteria, and susceptibility to stress. Presence of photosensitive porphyrins in the urine is diagnostic. Final diagnosis is made by measuring monopyrrole porphobilinogen deaminase in red blood cells. Although, the patient described above is suffering from acute intermittent porphyria, he remains in need of treatment for his acute psychosis. It is considered appropriate to employ traditional psychiatric medication for his immediate management. Psychotic patients and even elderly demented patients may well benefit from treatment with antipsychotics, even if the symptoms are of an organic cause. In general, small doses of a high-potency neuroleptic, such as haloperidol or risperidone may be used. Patients given these medications may exhibit extrapyramidal, hypothalamic, and antiadrenergic side effects. In addition, behavioral and environmental approaches, such as frequent reassurance and reorientation, reduction of distracting stimuli, or posey-type restraints with frequent nursing checks, should be used.

In a well-designed and important study at the ED of Harbor UCLA, 63 of 100 consecutive patients who presented with new-onset psychotic symptoms were found to have organic causes of their symptoms. One of the most striking findings in this study is that only 33 of the 63 patients would have been diagnosed by history and physical examination alone. At least 8 of the 63 patients would not have been diagnosed had they not had a CT scan or, in the presence of fever, a lumbar puncture. This should again remind physicians working in an ED that discriminating between organic causes of mental illness and non-organic causes is crucial. When the psychiatric symptoms have an organic cause and occur acutely, the term delirium is often used to describe the patient's status. The "WHHHHIMPS" mnemonic provides the health provider with a quick instrument for remembering most of the predominate life-threatening reversible causes of delirium.

Table 1. Causes of Delirium

W	Wernicke's encephalopathy
H	Hypoxia or hypoperfusion of CNS
H	Hypertensive encephalopathy
H	Hypoglycemia
H	Hypercalcemia
I	Intracerebral hemorrhage/Infection
M	Meningitis/encephalitis
P	Poisoning/Porphyria
S	Substances and drugs/Steroids

Even with limited historical information, the health provider may still have the ability to detect an organic from a non-organic cause of mental illness. Two clues to the presence of a delirium have been identified. First, the onset of the psychosis is generally quite abrupt, often occurring over the course of hours. Second, the symptoms associated with delirium often vary in intensity over time. An initially highly agitated and paranoid patient may be found to be reasonably calm and relatively coherent only a few hours later.

If the patient is unable to respond during the history often times friends or family members are able to provide the needed information. The interviewer conducting the history of a psychiatric patient should heed a few guiding principles: the patient should be removed from any current crisis situation or disturbing conditions, always be as honest with the patient as allowed by the situation, allow the patient the opportunity to speak, ask open ended questions, attempt to remain neutral and non-judgmental, and do not intimidate, argue, shout, or touch the patient.

When first attempting to discriminate between organic and functional illness, one should do a thorough general exam. The exam should focus on: affect, attention, memory, language and speech, visual/spatial orientation, and the patient's ability to understand concepts. A patient's orientation, especially to time of day is often very sensitive in diagnosing delirium. If the patient confuses the time of day (i.e. they believe it to be night when in actuality it's day), they should be considered delirious until proven otherwise. Disorientation generally accompanies impaired attention and immediate recall. Attention can be assessed my number recall. A normal person cannot hold a seven-digit phone number in short-term memory. A normal attention span allows for a six digits to be repeated in a forward fashion. In a crisis, a five-digit span is acceptable. Four or fewer digits suggest the need for a more thorough assessment. When asking these questions, the physician must be confident that a patient is attentive when testing a digit span, repeat the numbers slowly, and wait until they are finished before repeating the digits. Two or three tests are more accurate than a single trial.

A brief and directed mental status exam may further aid the emergency physician in determining the etiology of the mentally illness. The exam starts by observing the patient with particular attention paid to the general appearance and personal hygiene. A non-clean, unkempt or disheveled individual often signifies a long-term problem, but does not totally rule-out an organic component to the patient's presentation. Cognitive impairment discovered during the exam, strongly suggests a functional impairment. The patient's affect can also be quite helpful. Labile affects are often seen in mania whereas a blunted affect is often indicative of depressed or schizophrenic patients. Attention is determined by using serial 7s. Serial 7s are not used to establish intellectual function and the inability to attend may be indicative of a functional element. Delirious patients usually have difficulty with language and speech. Any form of aphasia suggests an organic etiology.

Delirious patients differ in the details of their illness from those patients with other psychiatric disorders. Delirious patients are generally disoriented, with an accompanying significant impairment in performing calculations and construction. They can have visual hallucinations and delusions, which are also common in patients with a presentation of psychosis. However, visual illusions are more suggestive of delirium. An example of a delirious illusion would be the patient who sees the form of their dead grandmother in a dark corner instead of a mop. The most common delusions accompanying delirium are paranoid delusions.

The text *Diagnostic and Statistical Manual of Mental Disorders fourth edition* (DSM IV) is considered the official diagnostic nomenclature and presents the criteria for mental health diseases. Published by the American Psychiatric Association, patients are diagnosed based on a framework of 5 separate axis's:

- axis I -clinical syndromes of mental disorder
- axis II -personality disorders, and developmental disorders,
- axis III - general medical conditions
- axis IV or V - psychosocial stressors and adaptive functioning.

SCHIZOPHRENIA

In addition to distinguishing delirium from non-organic mental illness, emergency medicine physicians must have a working knowledge of the common presentations of mental illness that are encountered in the emergency setting. An acute exacerbation of schizophrenia is a disease that is frequently treated in the emergency department. Overt signs of schizophrenia often first becomes manifest during adolescence or early adult life. According to the DSM IV a patient must exhibit two or more of the following symptoms: delusions, hallucinations, disorganized speech, grossly disorganized or catatonic behavior, and negative symptoms such as flattening of affect, poverty of speech, or an inability to perform goal-directed activities. Additionally, there must be a sharp deterioration from the patient's prior level of functioning (work, school, self-care, or interpersonal relations), and there must be continuous sign of disturbance (including prodromal symptoms) for at least 6 months. The positive symptoms are often predominately displayed by the patient speaking in a "word salad" or jumbled sentence fragments often with loose associations centered on bizarre or disorganized delusions. A brief discussion of the negative symptoms of schizophrenia is worthwhile. Although often less useful for developing a differential diagnosis, it may assist in the physicians approach to these patients. The negative symptoms mainly consist of flat affect, poverty of speech, or content of speech, and a reduction of expressive gestures. These symptoms can be produced by acute exacerbations of schizophrenia as well as depression or by typical antipsychotic medications.

Eugene Bleuler's four A's is an excellent tool to assist in remembering the symptoms of schizophrenia. The first A stands for auditory hallucination. The voices can be accusatory or commanding and are commonly in the third person ("John is no good"). Autism, the second Bleuler A, or loss of contact with reality is another symptom seen with schizophrenics. Autism is often represented as a breakdown of boundaries between the patient and the surrounding world. Schizophrenics believe that others can read or control their thoughts and often that their thoughts are being taken away or blocked. The third A represents an affect that is found to be inappropriate. The schizophrenic is often found laughing or becoming emotional at improper times. The final A stands for ambivalence. Schizophrenics often appear to lack interest in most of the outside world even in regards to their own care.

Schizoaffective disorder is separate issue from schizophrenia and is a rather difficult diagnosis to make without an adequate history. Indications may be found from the presence of psychotic symptoms consistent with schizophrenia, mixed with prominent affective symptoms. The key to the diagnosis is a history of psychotic symptoms in the absence of mood symptoms, which is often impossible to determine in an emergency setting.

As mentioned previously, the treatment of patients suffering from schizophrenic symptoms, either from an organic or non-organic cause can be very similar. Haldoperidol 5-10 mg every hour given intravenously, intramuscularly, or orally has been shown to be very effective in the acute and chronic treatment of patients demonstrating schizophrenic symptoms. Other antipsychotic medications, namely resperidol, have also been shown to be effective. The mechanism of action for antipsychotics is still not well understood, but it is known that drugs within this class act as dopamine antagonists. These medications can have effects in 1 hour after oral and 10-15 minutes after being given intramuscularly or intravenously. Combativeness can be calmed in 24-48 hours, negativism and withdrawal, delusions and hallucinations stopped in 2 weeks, and the patient often returns to his baseline mental status in 4-8 weeks. The antipsychotic medications are generally lipid soluble, detoxified by the liver, and are not addictive.

Neuroleptic malignant syndrome (NMS) is a rare, possibly lethal, and idiosyncratic disease that occurs at the onset of treatment with an antipsychotic. Generally, the potential to be affected by NMS increases when a second drug is introduced. Within 24-72 hours muscle rigidity, high temperatures of up to 42 degrees Celsius, and hypoventilation because of chest wall rigidity can be seen. Diphenhydramine 50 mg given intramuscular or intravenously is often used to treat any dystonia encountered after administering an antipsychotic.

Most schizophrenics require a sheltered environment to function adequately. It is of note that without medication 70% of schizophrenic patients will patients will relapse. The common reasons for medication non-compliance amongst schizophrenics are due to the patient being generally disorganized, a negativism towards the taking of medications, a fear of medications. Additionally, 5-25% of patients can not tolerate or do not respond to any certain medication. Restraints may be required, and a psychiatric consult is highly recommended to assist in treatment and the final patient disposition.

SECOND CASE STUDY

A 31-year-old man is brought to the ED by his wife. The wife tells you, that her husband had a vasectomy 1 month ago. Since that time, he has been chronically tired, suffering from insomnia, and has completely lost his appetite. What's your approach to this patient?

A physician should begin their approach to the patient above with a thorough a history and physical. Unless unadvisable, there should be discussions with individuals close to the patient to discover any further information in regards to general mood and attitudes the patient has been demonstrating lately. Important questions to ask of the patient at this time would include: "has your mood changed lately?," "have you been upset, angry, or nervous?", and "has your thinking been different in any way?" The previous example questions are open-ended and allow the patient to better define his symptoms. It is also important to ask about current suicidal or past suicide attempts or suicidal ideation. Questions regarding the use of drugs and alcohol may also provide useful information. Afterwards a complete physical exam, including a genital exam is appropriate. The next step may include laboratories, which would include a CBC searching for anemia and a set of standard chemistries paying close attention to glucose.

The patient above suffers from a mood disorder and in particular an adjustment disorder with a depressed mood. Vasectomies have been shown to be a frequent precursor of a postoperative depression, as are hysterectomies in the female. Sleep and appetite disturbances, lack of energy and tiredness are common manifestations of depression. Mood disorders are often found to include some combination of emotional, cognitive, somatic or behavioral symptoms; and can be classified as depressive or manic. Mood syndromes are considered clinically significant when symptoms become distressing or they begin to interfere with the patient's function in usual life roles.

Major depressive disorder is the most common psychiatric illness, with a lifetime prevalence of 17.1%. It is also the most common mood disorder seen in the ED setting. The presentation may be subtle and have the potential for lethality. The National Comorbidity Survey data demonstrated that the lifetime prevalence of affective disorders in the general population is 19.3% and the 1-year prevalence of affective disorders in the general population is and 11.3%. In comparison, the lifetime prevalence of any anxiety disorder is 24.9% and the 1-year prevalence of any anxiety disorder is 17.2%. Additionally, in a review of the clinical characteristics and diagnoses of 544 patients who visited one of four psychiatry emergency services (PESs) in Saskatoon, Canada, in a 3-month period in 1987 showed that 23.6% of patients suffered from affective disorders and 24.8% of patients suffered from anxiety disorders. This demonstrates that even in this specialized setting, mood and anxiety disorders are common.

A major depressive episode is characterized by a minimum of five of the following nine symptoms, including at least one of the first two, persisting for 2 weeks or longer, and leading to significant distress or functional impairment:

- depressed mood
- diminished
- hedonic capacity
- significant change in weight or appetite, insomnia or hypersomnia
- psychomotor agitation or retardation
- fatigue or loss of energy
- feelings of worthlessness or guilt
- diminished concentration or indecisiveness
- recurrent thoughts of death or suicide

More than 50% of patients with psychiatric illness will initially present with somatic complaints to primary care clinics. Of these patients, half fail to admit to depression or sadness when asked. These individuals will instead describe their mood as apathetic, anxious, or portray an inability to have or express emotions. When patients are willing to discuss their experiences they will often describe their emotional state as sad, blue, anxious, irritable or empty. Depression often creates a diminished capacity for enjoyment or lessened interest in all aspects of the patient's life, including work and loved ones. Cognitively, depression often creates a barrier to concentration or memory and can impair ones decision-making ability. It is common for those suffering with a depressive mood to express inappropriate guilt and to express feelings of worthlessness, hopelessness, or suicidal ideation.

Emergency physicians often encounter depressed mood patients in the ED because of the physical manifestations (imagined or real) of their disease. Complaints of unusual physical pain, gastrointestinal distress, fatigue, diminished energy, insomnia or hypersomnia as well as changes in appetite or weight, or decreased libido are commonly encountered by the physician. When performing the history and physical the physician should pay special attention to any psychomotor agitation or retardation, poor eye contact, tearfulness, long speech latency, minimal spontaneous speech, or poor vocal inflection. These behavioral characteristics can add evidence that the patient is suffering from a depressed mood and this may help steer the rest of the exam.

Patients with deep depression may be confused with schizophrenic patients because of the presence of delusions. Patients with mood disorders, however, tend to have delusions that are better organized and more coherent than those seen in schizophrenic patients. In addition, where schizophrenic patients often hear long-winded dialogue that involve more than one voice and in the third person, those with a mood-induced psychosis hear short verses, single voice and in the second person ("You are a terrible person "). There is a high potential for lethal consequences of mood syndromes such as behavioral problems, self-neglect, and self-destructive actions.

Although establishing a definitive diagnosis from the emergency setting is often not possible, the ED physician should attempt to collect detailed information. In this effort, it is it suggested to gather collateral information from family members, friends, outpatient treatment providers, or others with knowledge of the patient's history that may assist with diagnostic clarification. Attempts to provisionally classify depressed patients into a general category may aid in their final disposition. Depression can be a response to a stressful event, caused by a medical condition, a medication, or psychoactive substance. It can coexist with other psychiatric or medical disorders as well, or it may be difficult to find an underlying etiology.

It must be mentioned that more than 50% of individuals who experience a major depressive episode have a recurrence. Of these individuals with a recurrent episode, 15% of individuals with recurrence or severe major depression successfully commit suicide. When a patient is profoundly depressed they are more likely to be immobilized by the absolute depth of their depression. When beginning to recover from the depressive apathy, he or she is still profoundly depressed but is more mobile and active, and at that time are more likely to out their depression with suicide. When depression and other psychiatric disease coexist, the illness will often seem to be more severe. Comorbid depression and anxiety are associated with increased suicide risk, increased morbidity, poorer acute and long-term outcome, and increased treatment resistance. Schizophrenia also has a strong correlation with depression, with one-fourth of schizophrenics presenting with a depressed mood. The ultimate goal of EM physician should be behavioral control, medical screening, and psychiatric triage. Prolonged observation and evaluation in the emergency setting should be avoided. The treatment of depressed individuals in the emergency setting is extremely difficult without a thorough and reliable history. If a good history is obtained and the patient is believed to be at low-risk for self-injury, it is appropriate to send the patient home with observation by friends or family. The patient can also be placed on a low-dose antidepressant, which should be selected based on efficacy, side-effect profile, and lethality of overdose. All currently available antidepressants are of approximately equal efficacy.

Tricyclic antidepressants, with their significant side-effect burden, need for titration, and the risk for lethal overdose with a relatively small quantity, are a poor antidepressant choice from the emergency setting. The selective serotonin reuptake inhibitors and the serotonin norepinephrine reuptake inhibitors are less toxic in overdose and are generally better tolerated than the tricyclics. If there is concern for the patient's safety or a thorough history is unachievable a psychiatric consult should be obtained and admission must be considered.

MANIA

In addition to depression, mood disorders include mania. Manic patients are felt by many physicians to be the most difficult patient to contend with in the emergency setting. Acutely manic patients brought to the ED may require seclusion, restraint, or emergency pharmacologic intervention to ensure safety for patients, staff, and the public. The diagnosis of mania, according to the DSM IV, should include at least three of the following seven symptoms (four if mood is irritable):

- inflated self-esteem or grandiosity
- decreased need for sleep
- pressured speech
- racing thoughts or flight of ideas
- distractibility
- agitation or increased goal-directed activity
- excessive involvement in pleasurable activities with a high potential for severe consequences.

Mania is often initiated in predisposed patients by a physiologic or psychosocial stress or induced by somatic therapies, including antidepressants. Psychotic mania and the active phase of schizophrenia may be difficult to differentiate, especially if the mood is irritable or dysphoric. Manic patients can often be identified quickly in the ED by their wearing of bright clothing and their often unusual frenetic psychomotor activity or mood lability. Manic patients will often have a recent history of impulsivity and poor judgment. These individuals are known to speak with neologisms, clanging, rhyming, punning, or incomprehensible word salad. Delusions are present in approximately 75% of all manic patients. The lifetime risk for completed suicide is approximately 19%. In a community sample, 11% of individuals with mania were violent in the previous year. Rapid tranquilization, best achieved with a long acting benzodiazepine such as lorazepam, is often quickly required to help calm the acutely manic patient who is aggressive or at risk of injury to self or others. If tranquilization can be delayed, a low-stimulation environment has been demonstrated to assist in calming the manic patient. Afterwards, strict adherence to set limits creates a point of reference for the patient and will allow for an orderly exam of the patient.

Panic attack is the final topic to be discussed in this chapter. It is relevant to the practice of emergency medicine because of its commonality among patients visiting the ED. In one study conducted in an emergency psychiatric hospital, 25% of 544 patients received a diagnosis of a primary anxiety disorder. In a second study, 25% of 441 consecutive patients seen in an urban emergency department with a chief complaint of chest pain met the criteria for panic disorder. The National Comorbidity Study found a lifetime prevalence of panic disorder of 3.5%. The prevalence is higher among women than men and the young versus the old. In addition, there is a high correlation of comorbid psychiatric disorder and generalized anxiety disorder (GAD).

Panic attacks are sudden and discrete episodes that are marked by an overwhelming fear and a preponderance of physical symptoms. The somatic symptoms often include palpitations, tachycardia, and sweating and often present to the ED with the patients fearing that they are "dying" or "going crazy." The diagnosis of panic disorder, in the emergency setting, is often straightforward because these attacks are often recurrent, although unexpected. However, patients experiencing an initial panic attack episode can be quite concerned that they are going to die or that they are having a heart attack. Emergency physicians should not be duped by a well looking patient. It is common for patients, who recently suffered a panic attack, to have their symptoms completely resolve before being seen by the emergency physician. Patients presenting to the ED with symptoms consistent with panic attack should have a complete history and physical taken and anxiety should be the working diagnosis only when indicated. If the diagnosis of panic disorder is in question a more extensive work-up should be undertaken.

When examining patients in the midst of their attack, steps should generally be taken to decrease anxiety and to help reduce autonomic arousal. In the case of patients who appear to have completed their panic attack, anxiety over the return of symptoms is an important patient concern and may need to be urgently addressed. Controlled breathing techniques and redirecting the patient's attention from what is feared (e.g., heart attack or another panic attack) to what is actually happening (e.g., chest pain caused by hyperventilation) can often be very helpful. A study of patients with diagnosed panic disorder that received coronary angiography found that more than half of these patients who had normal coronary arterial flow on angiography stated that they were unable to work because of persistent symptoms. As is plainly seen, panic attack patients are often not reassured by negative information. Assessing spiritual needs; perception of support; common fears, such as isolation, helplessness, and mode of death; and other such psychological concerns are paramount to alleviating anxiety. When it is imperative to decrease the anxiety of the patient pharmacologic intervention is often necessary. A benzodiazepine with rapid onset and long duration, like Lorazepam, is effective and is available in both oral and parental forms. Beta-adrenergic blockers appear helpful when the anxiety is associated with stagefright, marked tremor and tachycardia. Finally, an interesting study on the treatment for panic disorder involved two groups of individuals suffering from panic disorder. In the first group, the exposure group, individuals were instructed to return to the situation as soon as possible after the interview and to wait there until the anxiety decreased. In the second group, patients only received reassurance. In the assurance group the frequency of panic attacks increased, and little difference was noted on objective measures of distress. In the exposed group panic attacks decreased in frequency and scores on the questionnaires improved significantly.

If it is believed that an organic cause with a psychotic component is responsible for the anxiety, haloperidol, 0.5 to 2 mg orally can be titrated every 2 hours to achieve relief.

A panic attack patient can most often return home after an acute episode. Self-injury is unlikely in patients with "pure" panic disorder. Often a short-course prescription for benzodiazepines is a good choice upon discharge. Care should be taken that medications are generally not given for more than 3-days. The patient may require a psychiatric consult, especially if there is little improvement over time or a comorbid psychiatric condition is thought to exist. Insisting upon quick follow-up for the patient will help ensure the patients long-term success.

REFERENCES

1. Lagomasino I, Daly R, Stoudemire A: Medical assessment of patients presenting with psychiatric symptoms in the emergency setting. *Psychiatr Clin North Am*, 1999, Dec; 22(4): 819-50, viii-ix.
2. Reeves RR; Pendarvis EJ; Kimble R Unrecognized medical emergencies admitted to psychiatric units. *Am J Emerg Med* - 01-Jul-2000; 18(4): 390-34.
3. Sulkowicz KJ: Psychodynamic issues in the emergency department. *Psychiatr Clin North Am* - 01-Dec -1999;22(4): 911-22
4. Richards CF; Gurr DE Psychosis. *Emerg Med Clin North Am* - 01-May-2000; 18(2): 253-62, ix
5. King PH; Petersen NE; Rakhra R; Schreiber WE Porphyria presenting with bilateral radial motor neuropathy:evidence of a novel gene mutation. *Neurology* - 9-Apr-2002; 58(7): 1118-217.
6. Schriger DL; Gibbons PS; Langone CA; Lee S; Altshuler LL: Enabling the diagnosis of occult psychiatric illness in the emergency department: a randomized, controlled trial of the computerized, self-administered PRIME-MD diagnostic system. *Ann Emerg Med* - 01-Feb-2001; 37(2): 132-40
7. Sanders AB. Missed delirium in older emergency department patients: a quality-of-care problem. *Ann Emerg Med*. March 2002;39:338-341.
8. Reeves RR; Pendarvis EJ; Kimble R Unrecognized medical emergencies admitted to psychiatric units. *Am J Emerg Med* - 01-Jul-2000; 18(4): 390-3
9. Murphy BA Delirium. *Emerg Med Clin North Am* - 01-May-2000; 18(2): 243-52
10. Diagnostic and Statistical Manual IV, ed 4. Washington, DC, American Psychiatric Association, 1994
11. Phenomenology and treatment of psychotic disorders in the psychiatric emergency service. Forster PL - *Psychiatr Clin North Am* - 01-Dec-1999; 22(4): 735-5413.
12. Möller A; Hell D The general psychological concept in the later work of Eugen Bleulers. Comparison with a summarized description from a forgotten theory 60 years after the final publication (1939)] Möller A - *Fortschr Neurol Psychiatr* - 01-Apr-1999; 67(4): 147-54
13. Blanchard JC; Curtis KM Violence in the emergency department. *Emerg Med Clin North Am* - 01-Aug -1999; 17(3): 717-31, viii
14. Geddes J, Freemantle N, Harrison P, Bebbington P. Atypical antipsychotics in the treatment of schizophrenia: systematic overview and meta-regression analysis. *Br Med J* 2000; 321(7273): 1371-1376.
15. Milner KK; Florence T; Glick RL Mood and anxiety syndromes in emergency psychiatry. *Psychiatr Clin North Am* - 01-Dec-1999; 22(4): 755-7717.
16. Moore JD; Bona JR Depression and dysthymia. *Med Clin North Am* - 01-May-2001; 85(3): 631-4418.
17. Merritt TC. Recognition and acute management of patients with panic attacks in the emergency department.*Emerg Med Clin North Am* - 01-May-2000; 18(2): 289-300

INTERNATIONAL EMERGENCY MEDICINE

John D. Cahill, M.D.[*]

What possible role does emergency medicine play in the international arena? This paper will discuss the numerous ways that the emergency medicine physician can contribute to international medicine. Emergency medicine physicians are well suited to work in international medicine for a variety of reasons. They have a broad knowledge of almost all aspects of medicine, excellent clinical skills, and work well under pressure. Our specialty and colleagues should remember that one does not necessarily have to go to remote corners of the world to make a difference.

EDUCATION

Education is one of the most important things that an emergency medicine physician can do. To date, there are only four countries that are considered to have developed emergency medicine: USA, Canada, Australia, and the United Kingdom. Therefore, the rest of the world is in need of understanding the concepts of emergency medicine. Many of the basic principles and practices of emergency medicine are easy to learn and applicable in any environment. Simple protocols and a basic understanding of resuscitative measures can save many lives. One does not need expensive and high tech equipment to make a difference. An example being the amount of mortality from diarrhea. In an emergency situation, diarrhea/dehydration may cause 25-50% of the deaths. A simple understanding of proper fluid resuscitation could significantly decrease this number. Another goal should be to help lay the foundation and infrastructure for proper training programs in emergency medicine.

Teaching overseas can be directed at an individual, institution, university, non government organization, or a government agency. One of the main objectives should be to instill some basic skills to students that allow them to pass these on to their other colleagues. Textbooks, videos, and the internet are other ways one can contribute. A simple video on neonatal resuscitation could be readily distributed throughout the world

[*] John D. Cahill, M.D., Assistant Professor of Community Health at Brown Medical School, Department of Emergency Medicine/Rhode Island Hospital, Department of Infectious Diseases/The Miriam Hospital, Providence, Rhode Island

and save many lives. Telemedicine is another field that will be expanding in the years to come. At home, one can also encourage exchange programs with other students, physicians, or other health care providers. Research is another mean to contribute, and can be based in basic science, diagnostic techniques, or clinical medicine.

DISASTER MEDICINE

Who better is prepared to be the expert in this field? One can focus on emergency preparedness or one of the aspects of disaster medicine:

- natural (ex: floods, earthquakes, volcanoes)
- manmade (ex: aviation accidents)
- terrorism (ex: biochemical, chemical, nuclear.)

TRAVEL/WILDERNESS MEDICINE

A variety of topics fall under this, including: high altitude medicine, diving medicine, maritime/cruiseship medicine, and evacuation services.

CONFLICT AND WAR

Conflicts and warfare around the globe continue to cause a demand for emergency physicians. One usually thinks of conventional war when thinking of conflict. However, there are very few wars fought in this nature. This type of warfare is high tech, expensive, and requires many resources to sustain it. In reality, most conflicts fall into one of 3 categories:

- fractionated
- genocide
- regional/state based

Fractionated warfare is the most common from of war for many reasons: it is cheap, opportunistic, small arms are readily available, there are often no clearly defined borders, and it can last for indefinite periods of time. Examples of fractionated warfare include "freedom fighters" or "guerilla warfare". Genocide is another form of low tech war which can be easily carried out. Propaganda can play a large role and once again this type of conflict can be sustained for long periods of time. There are many unfortunate examples of genocide, Rwanda being one. Regional conflicts are state based and rely on national armies or soldiers. Often they are centered around territorial or commercial gain. Here natural resources can play a role. They can also be based upon ethnicity. The continent of Africa is an unfortunate example, currently there are 17 regionally based conflicts occurring.

OUTCOMES

With direct combat, injuries can occur from: guns, knives, machetes, bombs, and other weapons. What one needs to remember are all the other outcomes associated with this problem. Although the list is long, several topics will be discussed here.

Loss of Infrastructure

This has a direct impact on almost all aspects of life. Hospitals may be destroyed, roads may be impassable, water lines may be broken, telephone services obsolete, and electricity cut off. The delivery of goods (food, medicine, and other supplies) may be stopped or significantly decreased. Therefore, inflation may occur on all goods. Making it even more of a challenge to feed one's family and obtain medicine. A secondary effect of this can be widespread violence, malnutrition, and disease.

Landmines

It is estimated that there 120 million active landmines on our planet, one for every 52 individuals. Over 90 countries are inflicted with landmines, with the continent of Africa having over 37 million. Landmines are very popular for many reasons: they are cheap (3-30 US dollars a piece), easy to deploy, and can remain active for up to 50 years. They allow for impassable borders to be set up for generations. Whether they are between countries, natural resources, or any targeted enemy or population. Not only do they cause bodily harm, but their economic impact can be devastating. Regions may become impossible to return home to or live in, agriculture becomes a dangerous activity, and transportation costs rise.

Often lower extremities receive the most damage from landmines, however the physician should remember that blast injuries can be described in one of three categories:

- primary: direct effect of blast overpressure on tissue
            lung
            ear: TM injury indicates significant force
            GI Tract
- secondary: objects fly through the air
            limbs
            penetrating trauma
- tertiary: people fly through the air

The average cost to treat an adult victim of a landmine is $3000 US dollars, including fitting for a prosthesis. Treating children is more problematic for several reasons, they often obtain more significant injuries and a new prosthesis needs to be fitted every 6-12 month as they are growing.

Displaced Populations

Often a population is forced to move due to the effects of war or conflicts: dangerous environment, political instability, lack of food: malnutrition, landmines, or disease to mention a few. Two populations to examine are refugees and internally displaced persons. A refugee is defined by the 1951 Convention relating to the Status of Refugees as "owing to a well founded fear of being persecuted for reasons of race, religion, nationality, membership of a particular social group, or political opinion, is outside the country of his nationality, and is unable to or, owing to such fear, is unwilling to avail himself of the protection of that country". It is estimated that there are at least 14.5 million refugees worldwide. Fortunately they have rights under international humanitarian law and are overseen by the United Nations High Commissioner for Refugees (UNHCR). It should be remembered that 2/3 of refugees are still living in a camp 5 years later. So long term planning and healthcare issues should be addressed.

Internally displaced persons (IDP's) are individuals who have been forced from their home, but remain within their national borders. This is a larger population with at least 25 million and growing. Sudan has the highest number at 4 million. Unfortunately, there is no single agency who is overall responsible for this population. These individuals are still under national jurisdiction and have a greater risk of persecution. Regardless of the population being served, there are many challenges that a physician faces. Some of the more important aspects will be reviewed.

THE EMERGENCY RESPONSE

Water

Water should be top priority in any emergency situation. It is the cornerstone of the foundation for an emergency response. Not only is water a necessity for life, but also for basic hygiene. In the initial response the quantity of water is more important than the quality. The absolute minimum requirement of water is 5 liters/person/day; this should be increased as soon as possible to reach a level of 15 – 20 liters/person/day. Other things to consider include:

- source of water
- accesibility to water
- location of water
- carrying containers for water
- protection of water

Water can be a source of disease on many different levels. Contaminated water as shown in table one contributes significantly to global morbidity and mortality. Freshwater can act as the home for the intermediate hosts that cause schistosomiasis and guinea worm infection. These infections commonly occur when an individual stands in water as they are collecting it. Lack of water or contaminated water can also contribute to trachoma which is a major cause of blindness or skin infections. Finally, water can act as the home to insect vectors that cause malaria, dengue fever, filariasis, onchocerciasis, and African trypanosomiasis.

Table 1: Water Borne from Fecal/Oral Ingestion

Disease	Morbidity Per Annum	Mortality Per Annum
Diarrhea	1,000 million	3.3 million
Typhoid	12.5 million	>125,000
Cholera	>300,000	>3000
Ascaris	1 billion	

Sanitation and Hygiene

Besides water, sanitation and hygiene are of top priority in the emergency response. It should be remembered that these measures are the first barrier to preventing the spread of fecal/oral disease. On average, the human produces 0.25 liters of stool/day and 1.5 liters of urine/day. One can easily see how quickly proper disposal and management of this can become a problem. When considering a sanitation system one needs to be culturally sensitive to the population that is being served. It is a futile effort to set up a sanitation system, if no one is going to use it. It is not a bad idea to involve the locals in setting up your system, thus avoiding some of these problems. Environmental implications should be considered as well: what impact may it have, how long is it going to be used, and is there any potential to contaminate the water supply? Sanitation system come in two forms as listed in table two. Also, one should also remember the old adage that our mother's told us "wash your hands"!

Table 2: Sanitation Systems

Wet	Dry
Water seal latrines	Trench
Aquaprives	Pit latrines
Oxfam Sanitation Unit	VIP latrine
	Bore holed
	Composting

Location

It cannot be stressed enough the importance of selecting a proper location. Ideally, the location should not be close to any border or place where fighting is taking place. It should not be on a significant grade. Accessibility is an important aspect: roads, trains, runways. Relief efforts become much more challenging if there is no way to deliver large amounts of goods. Security also needs to be carefully considered.

Food

Food stores come in either two forms: wet or dry. Things to carefully consider include: the manner that food is dispensed, who receives it, and how often. Protection of food stores as well is of importance. Nutritional assessment should be done, once the priorities of water, sanitation, and hygiene have been established. It should be remembered that not only do people die directly from malnutrition, but it predisposes to higher morbidity and mortality rates with existing disease. Vitamin A should be available, particularly when there is concern about measles.

Health

In the acute phase of an emergency the following diseases kill: malnutrition, diarrhea, pneumonia, measles, and malaria. Childhood vaccines should be readily available, particularly measles. Basic medicines should be stocked (one can refer to WHO list), intravenous fluids, and oral rehydration salts. After the initial acute phase of the emergency: geographic and population based diseases can be addressed. Some of more common communicable diseases contributing to morbidity and mortality include:

- Meningitis
- Hepatitis
- Viral Hemorrhagic Fevers
    Yellow Fever
    Dengue
    Other
- Japanese Encephalitis
- Typhus Fever
- Relapsing Fever
- Typhoid
- Influenza
- Leishmaniasis
- Plague
- African Trypanosomiasis
- Schistosomiasis
- Polio
- Tetanus
- Scabies
- HIV
- Tuberculosis

The spread of HIV can occur very readily in these situations for many different reasons. Lack of sterile medical equipment, tainted blood products, sexual activity, and the unavailability of condoms. Prostitution also significantly contributes to the spread of HIV. When people are desperate for food, supplies, or money, prostitution is a means to obtain them. Soldiers, truckers, and relief workers who are away from their significant other may engage in activities with prostitutes.

CONCLUSION

As long as mankind exists, there will be a need for physicians in the international arena to respond to crisis. Emergency medicine physicians are well suited for this response. Not only can we help the world, but our international efforts will gain further respect and acknowledgment for our specialty.

REFERENCES

1. Arnold JL., Introduction to International Emergency Medicine, *E Medicine*, 9/28/2001
3. Landmines, *International Committee of the Red Cross*, Geneva, Winter 2002
2. Convention and Protocol Relating to the Status of Refugees, *UNHCR/United Nations*, p 1-56
4. Eade D.,The OXFAM Handbook of Development and Relief, *OXFAM*, Oxford, March 1994, p22-33

INDEX

LaVergne, TN USA
01 April 2011
222632LV00005B/13/A